Cases of a

Doctor

Cases of a

HOLLYWOOD

Doctor

Edward Schwarz and Tomos Richards

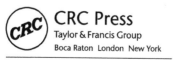

CRC Press
Taylor & Francis Group
Boca Raton London New York

CRC Press is an imprint of the
Taylor & Francis Group, an **informa** business

This book is dedicated to all of those staff working hard to keep our NHS free.

Contents

Contents

Preface

This book is designed for any medical student or junior doctor who finds revision a chore. It is not intended to be a comprehensive textbook or revision aid. It does not cover the whole medical curriculum. It does, however, contain many key concepts that are often taught in medical schools and on the wards and which frequently appear in exams. The book is intended to be readable and enjoyable to combat the dullness of your average textbook. A sort of medical 'toilet book'.

The book covers a wide range of conditions throughout the various specialities in medicine and surgery, from the basic to the more advanced. Cases are presented in anonymized format to preserve confidentiality and are laced with our attempts at humour. We hope you enjoy reading it, laughing at it and learning from it.

A proportion of our royalties will be donated to the mental health charity, Mind.

Ed Schwarz

Tom Richards

About the authors

Edward Schwarz MBBS FHEA

Ed is coming to the end of his GP training in Cornwall as an Educational Scholar. He graduated in 2011 from Peninsula Medical School (now Exeter Medical School and University of Plymouth Medical School), and completed his foundation years in Devon and Cornwall. He then moved to New Zealand for just under 2 years to work in a hospital, and it was there that he was inspired to write this book, with the aim of trying to make learning fun. Ed is also a Fellow of the Higher Education Academy.

Tomos Richards MBBCh MRCS

Tom is currently an Orthopaedic Trainee Registrar. After graduating from Cardiff University in 2011 he undertook his foundation and core training in Wales either side of a year working in New Zealand. He maintains a keen interest in medical education.

Acknowledgements

Figure 1.1 Adapted from Stiell IG, Wells GA, Vandemheen KL et al. (2001) The Canadian C-spine rule for radiography in alert and stable trauma patients. *JAMA* **286(15)**:1841–8.

Figures 3.1, 3.2 These tables are reproduced from the BTS/SIGN British guideline for the management of asthma by kind permission of the British Thoracic Society. British Thoracic Society (BTS)/Scottish Intercollegiate Guidelines Network (SIGN). British guideline on the management of asthma. Edinburgh: SIGN;2016 (QRG 153). Cited 4/2/2019. Available from URL: http://www.sign.ac.uk

Figure 6.2 National Institute for Health and Care Excellence (2014) Head injury, NICE clinical guideline 176. London: National Clinical Guideline Centre: www.guidance.nice.org.uk/guidance/CG176. NICE guidance is prepared for the National Health Service in England, and is subject to regular review and may be updated or withdrawn. NICE has not checked the use of its content in this publication to confirm that it accurately reflects the NICE publication from which it is taken.

Figure 6.1 Adapted from Teasdale G, Jennett B (1974) Assessment of coma and impaired consciousness. A practical scale. *The Lancet* **13;2(7872)**:81–4.

Figure 6.3 Image courtesy of Dr Ian Bickle, Radiopaedia.org, rID: 30036. Reproduced with permisison.

Figures 9.2, 11.1, 28.1, 28.2 ECGs courtesy of Life in the Fast Lane: https://lifeinthefastlane.com Reproduced with permission.

Figure 12.1 Adapted from Wells PS, Anderson DR, Rodger M et al. (2000) Derivation of a simple clinical model to categorize patients with a probability of pulmonary embolism: increasing the models utility with the SimpliRED D-dimer. *Thromb Haemost* **83**:416–20.

Figure 14.1 Adapted from Lip GY, Nieuwlaat R, Pisters R, Lane DA, Crijns HJ et al. (2010) Refining clinical risk stratification for predicting stroke and thromboembolism in atrial fibrillation using a novel risk factor-based approach: the euro heart survey on atrial fibrillation. *Chest* **137(2)**:263–72.

Figure 15.2 Adapted from the World Health Organization (1996) *Cancer Pain Relief, with a Guide to Opioid Availability. 2nd edn.* Geneva: WHO.

Figure 19.1 Image courtesy of Dr Andrew Dixon, Radiopaedia.org, rID: 10321 Reproduced with permission.

Figure 20.1 Image courtesy of Bobjgalindo: https://commons.wikimedia.org/wiki/File:Fluorescent_uric_acid.JPG), https://creativecommons.org/licenses/by-sa/4.0/legalcode

Figure 34.2 Clinical Assessment Tool. Courtesy of Dr Welch, Gloucestershire Clinical Commissioning Group, from 'The Big 6: Most Common Conditions Children Present with for Urgent Care'. Reproduced with permission.

Figure 41.1 Reproduced with permission from Lyme Disease Action: http://www.lymediseaseaction.org.uk

With special thanks to Jo Koster at CRC Press, Katy Nardoni from Cactus Design, and Peter Beynon. Special thanks also to Charlotte Richards, Clinical Pharmacist.

Abbreviations

ABCDE	Airway, Breathing, Circulation, Disability, Exposure (approach)
ABG	arterial blood gas
BMI	body mass index
BP	blood pressure
BTS	British Thoracic Society
BV	bacterial vaginosis
CCR	Canadian C-spine rule
CPR	cardiopulmonary resuscitation
CRP	C-reactive protein
CSF	cerebrospinal fluid
CT	computed tomography
CTPA	computed tomography pulmonary angiogram
DIC	disseminated intravascular coagulation
DIPJ	distal interphalangeal joint
DKA	diabetic ketoacidosis
DVLA	Driver and Vehicle Licensing Agency
DVT	deep vein thrombosis
ECG	electrocardiogram
FDP	flexor digitorum profundus
FDS	flexor digitorum superficialis
GCS	Glasgow Coma Scale
HDL	high-density lipoprotein
ICU	intensive care unit
LFT	liver function test
MRI	magnetic resonance imaging
NAI	non-accidental injury
NICE	National Institute for Health and Care Excellence
NSAID	non-steroidal anti-inflammatory drug
PE	pulmonary embolus
PEF	peak expiratory flow
RR	respiratory rate
RSV	respiratory synctival virus
SIGN	Scottish Intercollegiate Guidelines Network
TBSA	total body surface area
TIA	transient ischaemic attack

Cases by specialty

Note: there may be some overlap between cases and lots of them will be seen in primary care.

Cardiology
2, 28

Dermatology
13, 31

Emergency medicine
1, 6, 11, 23, 27, 39, 35, 36, 42

Endocrinology
7, 18, 21

Ear, nose and throat
24, 26

Gastroenterology
16, 22

Genetics
29

Haematology
5, 38

Infectious diseases
41, 43

Neurology
4, 14, 30

Non-clinical skills
32, 47

Opthalmology
51

Paediatrics
19, 34, 37

Psychiatry
33

Renal
9

Respiratory
3, 8, 12, 45, 46

Rheumatology
20

Sexual health
40, 50

Trauma and orthopaedics
10, 15, 17, 25, 44, 48, 49

Vascular
52

CASE 1

Humpty Dumpty is brought in to see you following a fall. His friends report that he was sitting on a 2 metre wall when he fell backwards. He has been drinking heavily. He immediately complained of neck pain and has not walked since the fall. He was alert at the scene and is otherwise fit and well and takes no regular medication.

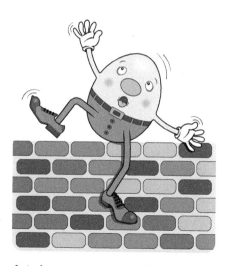

He is brought in by the paramedics on a stretcher, with his neck immobilized. On examination in the emergency department, he is in a lot of pain. He has grazes to his chin. He says his neck is hurting and you elicit cervical spine tenderness. You also notice bruising around his eyes and, on examining his ear, clear fluid draining on the right side.

i. What is the Canadian C-spine rule to aid in assessment of neck injuries?

The Canadian C-spine rule (CCR) is a useful guide to help decide whether imaging is required for suspected cervical spine injuries. It should be applied in alert and stable trauma patients only. CCR is only a tool and if there is any doubt, the clinician should have a low threshold for imaging. Plain radiographs can be used and if there is still uncertainty, a CT should be arranged. The chart overleaf (Fig. 1.1) illustrates this guide.

ii. Would this patient require further imaging of his neck?

In this instance, the patient would require further imaging as he fulfils several of the criteria for imaging, with a suspicion of cervical injury. He also would require further imaging of his head (see below).

iii. Given your examination findings (bruising around the eye and ottorhoea), what is this suggestive of?

This clinical picture is highly suggestive of a base of skull fracture and given this and his neck injuries, it would be prudent to image his head and neck at the same time, using CT to give a detailed and accurate picture.

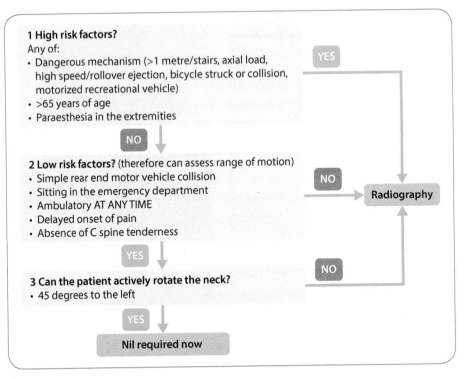

1 High risk factors?
Any of:
- Dangerous mechanism (>1 metre/stairs, axial load, high speed/rollover ejection, bicycle struck or collision, motorized recreational vehicle)
- >65 years of age
- Paraesthesia in the extremities

YES

NO

2 Low risk factors? (therefore can assess range of motion)
- Simple rear end motor vehicle collision
- Sitting in the emergency department
- Ambulatory AT ANY TIME
- Delayed onset of pain
- Absence of C spine tenderness

NO

Radiography

YES

NO

3 Can the patient actively rotate the neck?
- 45 degrees to the left

YES

Nil required now

Figure 1.1.

Base of skull fractures are uncommon; however, they are a favourite question to ask in exams due to their classical clinical signs:

- Battle's sign – bruising behind the ear, over the mastoid process of the temporal bone.
- Rhinorrhea or otorrhoea (due to CSF leakage).
- 'Racoon' eyes – bruising around the eyes.

OUTCOME

Humpty Dumpty underwent a full trauma CT scan. The images showed highly comminuted fractures of his thin shell-like cranium with intracerebral bleeding. The radiologist confirmed that he actually has no neck. He was transferred to the specialist trauma centre at King's; however, all of their men were unable to save him and he passed away later that day.

CASE 2

In the run up to Christmas, Mr S Claus, 72, books in for a 'Well Man' check-up. He does not come to the doctor that often as he says he is too busy, especially at this time of the year with his work as a delivery driver. On general questioning, he says he has been quite stressed recently given a number of factors. His elves have recently been on strike, citing health and safety concerns with the icy cold conditions. The postal workers strike has resulted in a delay in childrens' wish lists arriving to him and the Brexit vote has

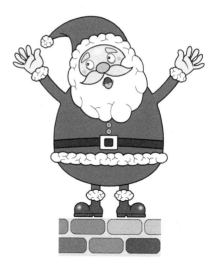

provided uncertainty with regards to visa issues with his worldwide travels. He admits to enjoying a glass or two of sherry, adding up to approximately 14 units per week, and mince pies and says his weight is a problem. He is fairly active, climbing up and down chimneys. On examination, his BP is 155/90 and his BMI is 32.8 (height 178 cm, weight 104 kg). The rest of his examination is normal. General screening bloods were also normal apart from a raised cholesterol:HDL ratio of 7.

i. What is a QRISK2 score, and how is it calculated?

The QRISK2 score is a validated scoring system recommended by NICE to assess cardiovascular risk over ten years. (There is now a QRISK3 score [2018] but it is not recommended by NICE.) It is used in primary prevention, therefore cannot be used in patients with coronary artery disease, or previous stroke and TIA, and takes into account the following variables: age; sex; BP; BMI; cholesterol/HDL ratio; whether a patient has diabetes; smoking status; ethnicity; a family history of coronary heart disease in a first-degree relative under the age of 60; deprivation (based on postcode); whether a patient is on treatment for BP; rheumatoid arthritis, chronic kidney disease, atrial fibrillation (due to their associated risk).

There are many online calculators to assist in calculation of the QRISK score.

ii. This patient has a QRISK2 score of 23%. What should be discussed with the patient?

A QRISK2 score of 23% means that based on population data, 23 out of 100 people with the same risk factors as the patient will likely have a stroke or a heart attack in the next ten years. Recent guidelines suggest that patients with a risk of more than 10% should be offered a statin.

iii. How should his blood pressure be managed?

This gentleman should be offered ambulatory BP monitoring. The patient has a BP monitor fitted, usually over 24 hours, that records BP at set intervals. This gives a better idea of the average BP and avoids 'white coat hypertension'. White coat hypertension is a phrase used to describe an elevated BP due to anxiety around seeing a doctor (from the days of wearing a white coat) that does not represent a true picture of the patient's overall readings If the ambulatory BP is persistently high, treatment options in this gentleman would include a calcium channel blocker (e.g. amlodipine) initially. Mr Claus also needs general advice including weight loss, cutting down alcohol and improving his diet.

OUTCOME

Mr Claus carefully considered the discussions during the consultation and decided not to start a statin or BP tablet. Instead, he made significant lifestyle changes and Mrs Claus strictly monitored his diet. He swapped mince pies for the carrots that were left for his reindeers. To help maintain his new lifestyle he decided to give up his delivery work stating that families would 'have to sort their own kids out'.

CASE 3

A 24-year-old big bad wolf presents to the emergency department in an ambulance. The crew report that he was found next to a pile of sticks and straw. A pig had called 999 from the safety of his stone house but had not helped as he was concerned for his own safety. Police were on the scene. The patient was struggling to breathe and apart from some inhalers, cigarettes and a packet of pork scratchings in his pockets, there was no other history from the patient. A passer-by said he had sounded very wheezy when exhaling.

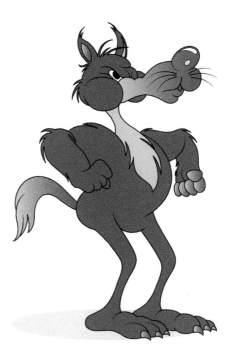

On examination in the emergency department, he is unable to talk in complete sentences. His oxygen saturations are 93%, his heart rate is 112, his respiratory rate is 29 and he is afebrile. He has widespread wheeze and his chest sounds tight. His BP is 104/98. He is alert but looks tired. You suspect a diagnosis of asthma.

i. What is the severity of this gentleman's asthma?

Assessing the severity of asthma is a favourite question of examiners and is also clinically useful, as it should be remembered that patients with severe asthma are at risk of death and those with mild to moderate asthma are at risk of deteriorating further. This gentleman would fit the criteria for acute severe asthma, as shown in Fig. 3.1. However, the fact that he is looking tired is a worrying sign.

ii. What is the immediate treatment?

After your assessment, following the ABCDE approach as per the UK Resuscitation Guidelines, high-flow oxygen should be applied to this patient as he is hypoxic. Nebulizers should be given immediately and can be given 'back to back' (2.5–5 mg salbutamol). Nebulized ipratropium bromide (500 μg 4 hourly) can also be used. Although steroids should be given as early as possible, remember that it will be several hours before they will be effective. If there is any evidence of infection, antibiotics should also be given.

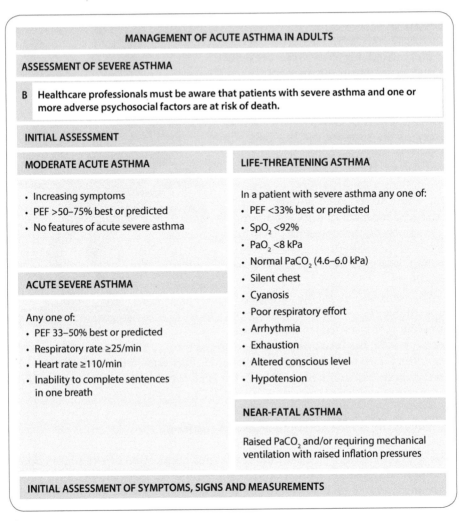

MANAGEMENT OF ACUTE ASTHMA IN ADULTS

ASSESSMENT OF SEVERE ASTHMA

B   Healthcare professionals must be aware that patients with severe asthma and one or more adverse psychosocial factors are at risk of death.

INITIAL ASSESSMENT

MODERATE ACUTE ASTHMA

- Increasing symptoms
- PEF >50–75% best or predicted
- No features of acute severe asthma

ACUTE SEVERE ASTHMA

Any one of:
- PEF 33–50% best or predicted
- Respiratory rate ≥25/min
- Heart rate ≥110/min
- Inability to complete sentences in one breath

LIFE-THREATENING ASTHMA

In a patient with severe asthma any one of:
- PEF <33% best or predicted
- SpO_2 <92%
- PaO_2 <8 kPa
- Normal $PaCO_2$ (4.6–6.0 kPa)
- Silent chest
- Cyanosis
- Poor respiratory effort
- Arrhythmia
- Exhaustion
- Altered conscious level
- Hypotension

NEAR-FATAL ASTHMA

Raised $PaCO_2$ and/or requiring mechanical ventilation with raised inflation pressures

INITIAL ASSESSMENT OF SYMPTOMS, SIGNS AND MEASUREMENTS

Figure 3.1.

iii. What would prompt a referral to intensive care?

According to the latest guidelines from the BTS, several factors would prompt a referral to the ICU (Fig. 3.2).

In this case, the patient looking tired is a worrying sign that he is deteriorating and senior help with anaesthetic support may be required. Following a recent coroner's inquest, Health Education England have issued recommendations, including that all doctors should familiarize themselves with 'Why Asthma Still Kills', published by the Royal College of Physicians.

REFERRAL TO INTENSIVE CARE

Refer any patient:

- Requiring ventilatory support
- With acute severe or life-threatening asthma, who is failing to respond to therapy, as evidenced by:
  - Deteriorating PEF
  - Persisting or worsening hypoxia
  - Hypercapnia
  - ABG analysis showing ↓ pH or ↑H⁺
  - Exhaustion, feeble respiration
  - Drowsiness, confusion, altered conscious state
  - Respiratory arrest

Figure 3.2.

OUTCOME

The patient improved with the treatment given and was discharged with a short course of high-dose steroid. He was reviewed by the practice asthma nurse and offered smoking cessation. He was issued with a restraining order forbidding him to go within 100 metres of the pig's home. He has since become a vegetarian.

CASE 4

A local pirate is brought in by ambulance to your emergency department. He has recently returned from a sailing holiday in the Caribbean. He is accompanied by another crew member, who smells strongly of rum. On questioning, he is not able to hold a conversation and he believes himself to be aboard his ship, 'The Jolly Roger.' He is able to follow commands, although rambles about travelling to the far end of the world.

On examination, he has a faint smell of rum on his breath, he is unkempt and has numerous tattoos on his arms. You perform a neurological examination and notice that on looking to the right, he gets double vision and his right eye does not appear to move (Fig. 4.1). You complete the neurological examination and as he walks out to the bathroom, you notice that he staggers from side to side with a wide-based gait, knocking over the notes trolley.

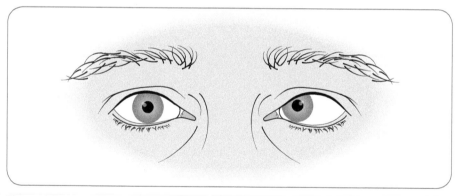

Figure 4.1.

i. Given this history, what is the most likely diagnosis?

The image demonstrates a sixth (abducens) cranial nerve palsy. When the patient tries to look to the right, the right eye fails to turn to the side. The triad of ophthalmoplegia, ataxia and confusion is classic for Wernicke's encephalopathy. Wernicke's encephalopathy is a neurological complication that results from a thiamine deficiency. Thiamine is a cofactor for several enzymes important in metabolism. It is needed more in times of high metabolic demand and high glucose intake. All three symptoms may not necessarily be present, resulting in underdiagnosis of this condition. This condition is more common in alcoholics due to malnourishment; however, Wernicke's encephalopathy can also occur in refeeding and dialysis patients.

ii. What is the treatment of this condition?

Because this condition is a result of thiamine deficiency, it is necessary to replace thiamine levels. Diagnosis is mainly made clinically and so high suspicion and opportunistic treatment of patients at risk should occur. It can be given intravenously acutely on admission and then patients can take oral thiamine. As it is needed most during periods of high glucose intake, doctors should avoid giving intravenous glucose without supplementation in an at-risk patient, as this may precipitate Wernicke's.

iii. What happens if this condition is left untreated?

If left untreated, the patient may go on to an irreversible condition known as Korsakoff's syndrome where there is marked retrograde and anterograde amnesia. The patient often confabulates. An example of confabulation would be a plausible sounding statement that cannot be true, such as, 'I fought in World War Two in the Welsh Guards,' yet the patient would have been only 5 years old at the time.

OUTCOME

The patient received intravenous B vitamin and thiamine complex on the ward and was given a prescription for thiamine tablets. He did not comply with his medication and continued to confabulate about buried treasure. He is frequently seen in the local park digging holes under trees and talking to birds.

CASE 5

Count Dracula, a 55-year-old man, is transferred from the nurse-led Day Case Unit to the emergency department. He was receiving a transfusion as he was found to be anaemic and was given one unit of blood group A. He appears confused and aggressive and has been trying to bite members of staff.

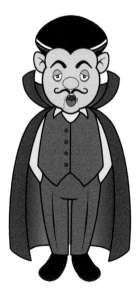

On careful examination the patient looks pale, has a temperature of 39.2°C, is itching and has a widespread urticarial rash. As you go to get intravenous access, he suddenly goes quiet and you notice his BP dropping. You resuscitate him with fluids and he is transferred to the ICU for inotropic support. His blood group is discovered to be group O. His haemoglobin is 73 g/L and his platelets are 25 ×10^9/L.

i. What blood group can this patient receive?

Group O is the universal donor group and this blood can be given to all patients. However, group O patients can only receive blood from other group O patients. AB group is the universal recipient group. The flow chart (Fig. 5.1) shows the different blood groups and their recipients. For example, group A patients can receive blood from group O or group A people, but they can only give blood to other group A or group AB patients.

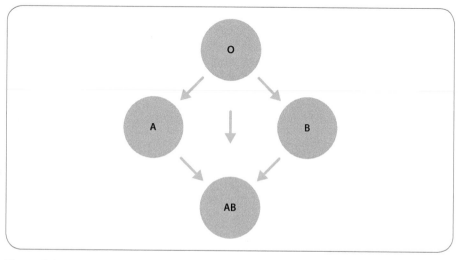

Figure 5.1.

There are also lots of other components to matching blood products, including rhesus groups. Giving the wrong blood group to a patient will result in an acute haemolytic reaction. The early signs of this are hypotension, fever, chest pain and, later, disseminated intravascular coagulation (DIC), causing generalized bleeding. Fortunately, this is a rare occurrence of about 1 in 35,000 transfusions and can happen during the first few millilitres of an infusion.

A less severe reaction that patients may develop is a febrile non-haemolytic reaction to blood products. This may be caused by cytokine release and normally resolves within 30 minutes and can be treated with paracetamol.

ii. How can you minimize an acute haemolytic reaction?

The majority of these events are caused by human error and they have been declared a Never Event in the UK. Patients should all have patient identifying bands on their wrists and blood bottles should be labelled at the bedside, confirming visually and verbally patient details. When giving the blood products, two trained healthcare professionals should again check the blood with the form and the patient. If there are any concerns during transfusing, the infusion should immediately be stopped.

iii. What do the patient's low platelets suggest?

This man may well be developing DIC where the clotting cascade is activated, causing clots to form in small vessels and bleeding.

OUTCOME

The patient unfortunately deteriorated further and was declared dead later that evening by the Foundation doctor on the ICU. He was transferred overnight to the morgue. The next day when the registrar went to complete the certification of death and cremation forms, there was no trace of the body or the mortuary staff other than a few blood spatters and some bat droppings on the floor.

CASE 6

JB, a 34-year-old man, is brought to the emergency department by a group of fishermen. He was found face down in the Mediterranean Sea and was unresponsive on being rescued from the water 4 hours ago. On arrival in the department he is combative and agitated. He has several passports with different identities on his person. On assessment he is maintaining his airway with no respiratory or circulatory disturbance. His observations are normal. He is able to obey your commands and he watches you when you speak; otherwise his eyes are closed. He is not sure where he is and keeps talking about a safe deposit box. He cannot remember what happened to him more than a few days before he was found. There is some bruising over his left temporal region and a small subcutaneous lump over his right shoulder.

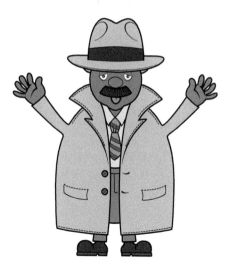

i. What does the patient score on the Glasgow Coma Scale?

The Glasgow Coma Scale (GCS) is a method of objectively measuring a patient's consciousness level. This patient's GCS score would be eyes 3, voice 4 and motor 6 = 13/15. The GCS score is calculated on a best possible score from eye opening, verbal response and motor response. It is scored from 3 to 15 as shown in Fig. 6.1.

Glasgow Coma Score		
Eye opening response	Spontaneously	4
	To voice	3
	To pain	2
	No response	1
Verbal response	Orientated	5
	Confused	4
	Inappropriate words	3
	Inappropriate sounds	2
	No response	1
Motor response	Obeys commands	6
	Localizes to pain	5
	Withdraws from pain	4
	Abnormal flexion	3
	Abnormal extension	2
	No response	1

Total score out of 15. Normal is 15. A comatose patient will have a score of 8 or less and a totally unresponsive patient will have a score of 3. Note 3 is the lowest possible score.

Figure 6.1.

It is useful to repeat the score in patients with a fluctuating consciousness level. An abridged tool sometimes used is the AVPU score (Alert, Voice, Pain, Unconscious). It is bad if you 'are in the PU' and senior help should be sought.

ii. What is the next appropriate management step?

NICE guidelines (**Fig. 6.2**) recommend urgent CT scanning of the head for the indications shown. This patient's GCS score is 13 at 4 hours post being found, and therefore he should proceed for urgent CT.

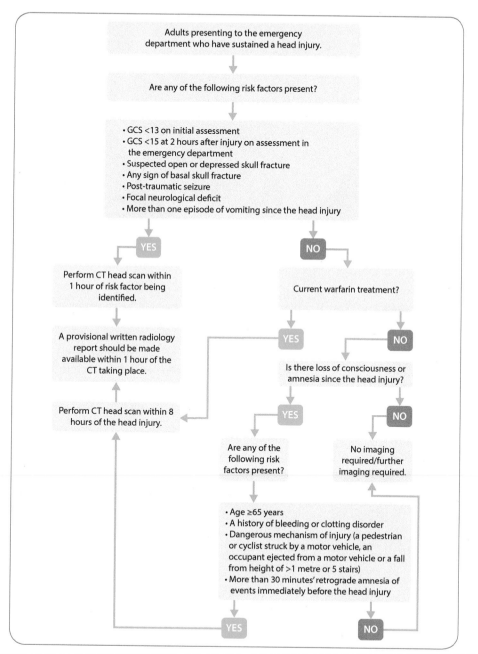

Figure 6.2.

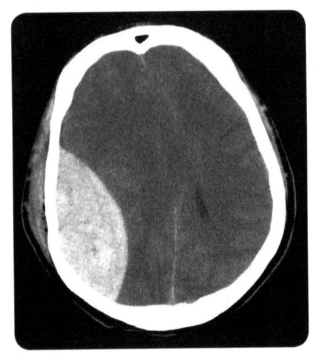

Figure 6.3.

iii. What does his CT scan show (Fig. 6.3), and what would be the management?

The CT scan shows a right-sided extradural haematoma. This a characteristically biconvex high intensity on non-contrast CT as bleeding is bound by the attachment of the dura to the suture lines. It is often caused by bleeding from the middle meningeal artery after trauma. The patient would need urgent discussion with a neurosurgeon with a view to proceeding for urgent evacuation of the haematoma.

OUTCOME

The patient underwent decompressive craniectomy and made a good postoperative recovery. He continues to have significant amnesia, although has regained many of his hobbies such as hand to hand combat and evasive driving. The swelling over his right shoulder was found to be a small metal foreign body that he had removed in the private sector.

CASE 7

A 12-year-old girl is brought to the emergency department by the local priest with repeated vomiting and abdominal pain occurring during an attempted exorcism. On questioning she has been very thirsty and drinking lots over the past week. They report her behaviour to have been bizarre with some inappropriate swearing and some self-harm to her abdomen. She has also had polyuria and reportedly urinated on the floor. On examination she appears confused and lethargic and has dry mucous membranes. After a full examination you take some blood tests (Fig. 7.1).

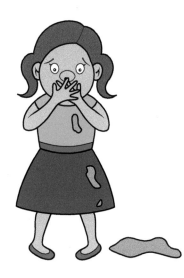

Hb	133 g/L	K	4.6 mmol/L
WCC	15.5 ×10⁹/L	Urea	11.9 mmol/L
Platelets	234 ×10⁹/L	Creatinine	98 µmol/L
Na	140 mmol/L	Glucose	34 mmol/L

Figure 7.1.

i. What is a normal blood sugar level?

Normal blood sugars are 4.0–5.4 mmol/L when fasting and up to 7.8 mmol/L 2 hours after eating (Fig. 7.2).

Plasma glucose	Normal	Prediabetes	Diabetes
Random	<11.1 mmol/L		>11.1 mmol/L
Fasting	<5.5 mmol/L	5.5–6.9 mmol/L	>7.0 mmol/L
2 hour after food	<7.8 mmol/L	7.8–11 mmol/L	>11.0 mmol/L

Figure 7.2.

ii. What is the likely diagnosis, and what other biochemical investigations are likely to be abnormal?

The blood tests (Fig. 7.1) show a significantly elevated blood glucose consistent with an untreated diabetic patient. In this presentation this suggests diabetic ketoacidosis (DKA). Venous gas analysis showed a metabolic acidosis and urinary and plasma ketones were present, confirming the diagnosis.

iii. How would you manage this patient?

DKA causes significant dehydration through the osmotic effect of elevated glucose. Fluid resuscitation is important to correct life-threatening dehydration before starting an insulin infusion to normalize blood glucose levels. In the past, large volumes of fluid were given intravenously but there is concern that this can potentiate cerebral oedema. Insulin drives potassium into cells, therefore potassium supplementation will be required alongside ongoing fluid replacement. Most hospitals now have protocols to standardize the management of DKA and the patient should be closely monitored in a high dependency unit or ICU. Once stable the patient will need full diabetic education and management to prevent further recurrences.

OUTCOME

The family of the patient were not happy with her management and she self-discharged when she was a bit more stable under the care of the Church. She was later reported as having been cured by the priests there.

CASE 8

A patient presents who is a 40-year-old widower. His son was also killed along with his wife in distressing circumstances. He presents to your emergency department via chariot from the local stadium. He had been fighting prior to him suddenly collapsing and there is no further information to be gleaned.

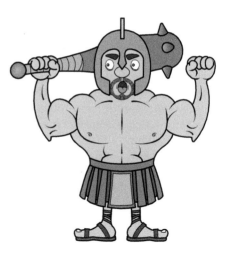

On examination he is alert and oriented with saturation of 85% on air. His respiratory rate is 38, heart rate 125, BP 110/70. He has reduced air entry in the right-hand side of his chest and you think he is hyperresonant on percussion. You notice a small stab wound to his right side. He is taken straight to resus and a chest radiograph is obtained (Fig. 8.1).

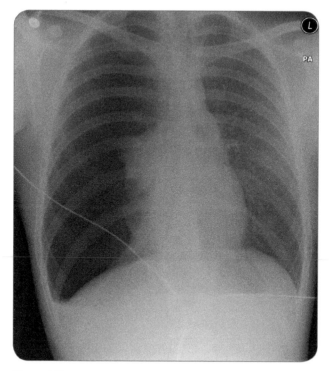

Figure 8.1.

i. What does the chest radiograph show?

The radiograph shows a right-sided pneumothorax evidenced by absence of lung markings and a darker appearance compared with the left. The trachea is central and not deviated. There is some flattening of the right hemidiaphragm.

As you obtain intravenous access, the patient's monitor starts beeping. On re-examination the patient has no pulse, is not breathing and there are no signs of life. You begin CPR on the patient and the cardiac arrest call is put out. While CPR is underway you try and remember the four H's and four T's (eight reversible causes of cardiac arrest) from your resuscitation course.

ii. What are the four H's and four T's?

These are designed to help resuscitation providers identify potential reversible causes. The four H's are Hypoxia, Hypovolaemia, Hypothermia and Hyper/hypokalaemia (and other metabolic causes including hypoglycaemia). The four T's are Tamponade, Tension pneumothorax, Toxins and Thromboembolic disease.

You do a quick examination of the patient while CPR is taking place and notice that there is no air entry on the right-hand side during ventilation. His trachea is also deviated to the left.

iii. What is the likely diagnosis, and what is the treatment?

A penetrating injury like this should raise suspicion of a tension pneumothorax. A tension pneumothorax is the progressive build up of air in the pleural space, normally due to a lung laceration or an open sucking chest wound acting as a one-way valve. Air can enter the pleural space but does not escape, increasing the intrathoracic pressure on that side and pushing the mediastinum to the opposite side. This may in turn obstruct the venous return to the heart, causing circulatory arrest. A needle thoracostomy should be performed. This would be in the second intercostal space, midclavicular line using a large cannula. This is only a temporizing measure and it would be necessary to position a chest drain in the safe triangle of the sixth intercostal space, midaxillary line and border of pectoralis major as a definitive treatment. Needle thoracostomy is not without its risks and should only be performed when absolutely necessary. However, in the case of circulatory collapse it is potentially lifesaving.

OUTCOME

The patient unfortunately did not survive from his wounds. Despite the best efforts of the local emperor to demonize him, a large state funeral was attended by large numbers of the public. His story was documented in a blockbuster movie production, which unfortunately glamourized the knife violence problem in modern culture.

CASE 9

A rectangular talking sponge is brought into the emergency department by a friend. He has been living in a discarded fruit under the sea for some time but has recently moved house to a rented flat on dry land. His friend has noticed him becoming increasingly lethargic since the move and he has been passing very dark urine. You assess him and notice he is very dry with reduced skin turgor. His heart rate is 120 bpm and BP is 93/60 mmHg. You order some blood tests (Fig. 9.1).

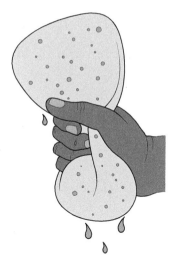

Na	148 mmol/L
K	6.5 mmol/L
Ur	18.4 mmol/L
Cr	246 μmol/L

Figure 9.1.

i. What are the causes of acute kidney injury?

They can be broadly classified into pre-renal, renal and post-renal causes. Pre-renal causes affect the perfusion pressure of the kidney and are often systemic (e.g. hypovolaemia from bleeding or diarrhoea and vomiting, sepsis or cardiac failure). Renal causes affect the cells of the kidney itself (e.g. glomerulonephritis, nephrotoxic drugs [e.g. gentamycin] or rhabdomyolysis). Post-renal causes result from obstruction and back-pressure on the kidney from pathologies such as ureteric stones, prostate hypertrophy or tumours.

ii. What ECG findings are associated with hyperkalaemia?

Hyperkalaemia can be precipitated by acute kidney injury. Abnormalities include peaking of T waves, widening of the QRS complex, prolonged PR interval and flattening of P waves. This progresses to produce a 'sine wave' appearance of the ECG and then cardiac arrest. An example ECG is shown (Fig. 9.2).

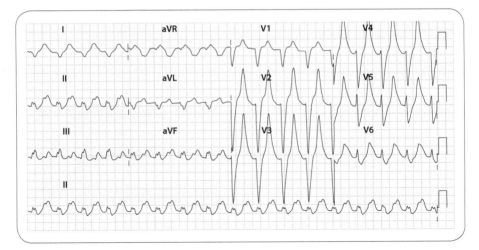

Figure 9.2.

iii. What is the management of hyperkalaemia?

Immediate management is via the ABC approach to the patient. Ten mL of 10% calcium gluconate should be given immediately intravenously to help stabilize the myocardium. Measures to drive potassium intracellularly include insulin and glucose (10 units Actrapid® with 50 mL 50% glucose) and salbutamol nebulizers. Definitive treatment is required by treating the precipitating cause, discontinuing any contributory medications (e.g. ACE inhibitors and spironolactone), and occasionally dialysis is required. In this case, treatment of the acute kidney injury through catheterization, intravenous fluid resuscitation with monitoring of input/output and avoidance of nephrotoxic medication may lead to a resolution.

OUTCOME

After full treatment as above the patient regained his robust spongy form and felt much better. He was strongly advised to remain in his marine environment to prevent any further 'drying out' episodes. Despite this, the strong allure of the beach party lifestyle was too much and he was readmitted 2 months later following a full moon party all night binge and required haemodialysis and a 2-week ICU stay.

CASE 10

A local teacher and explorer presents to your clinic complaining of some pain in his right hand. He reports having recently returned from an expedition in Egypt where he admits to using a whip repeatedly over a period of several weeks. He is normally fit and well other than a strong phobia of snakes. He denies any fever or wrist swelling. He complains of numbness and tingling in his thumb, index and middle finger. He reports this is worse at night and sometimes shaking his hand tem-

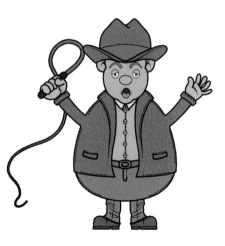

porarily improves the pain. On examination, he is afebrile. His hand does not look swollen or red. He does indeed have sensory loss over his thumb and index finger on the palmar side of his hand.

i. What is the most likely diagnosis?

The most likely diagnosis is carpal tunnel syndrome. This is caused by compression of the median nerve as it passes in the carpal tunnel under a fibrous ligament, the flexor retinaculum. Compression of this nerve results in pins and needles and numbness over the distribution described below. In more severe cases, there may be muscle weakness in the median nerve-innervated muscles of the thumb. It is more common in women, hypothyroidism, pregnancy, obesity and diabetes. Tasks involving repetitive and forceful motions may play a part in this condition, although this is still disputed. The dermatomal distribution of the nerves of the hand is shown (Fig. 10.1).

ii. How can you clinically confirm this diagnosis?

Examination may reveal wasting of the thenar eminence muscle bulk and altered sensation in the supplied fingers. Tinel's sign, which is tapping over the nerve at the flexor retinaculum, may elicit the paraesthesia in the hand. Flexing the wrist gently and then holding the wrist in this position is known as Phalen's manoeuvre, and if symptoms are reported by the patient, then this also suggests carpal tunnel syndrome. Nerve conduction studies are often performed to confirm the diagnosis.

iii. Which muscles of the hand does this nerve supply?

This is for some reason a favourite question in exams! They can be remembered by the pneumonic LOAF – **L**ateral lumbricals, **O**pponens pollicis, **A**bductor pollicis brevis and **F**lexor pollicis brevis.

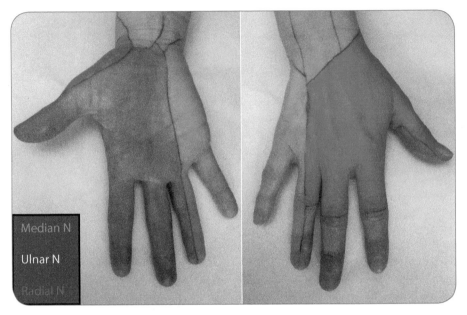

Median N

Ulnar N

Radial N

Figure 10.1.

OUTCOME

The patient wore a wrist splint that helped the symptoms and was referred for a carpal tunnel decompression via the local orthopaedic surgeon. He was unable to attend his scheduled outpatients appointment as he was on an archeological field trip, which was prolonged due to unexpected complications. When he finally returned he decided to go private after coming into a large sum of money from a local historical artefact collector.

CASE 11

A mass casualty scenario is rung through to your emergency department. A ship has hit an iceberg and heavy casualties are expected, with many patients having been submerged in the freezing cold North Atlantic Sea. A 25-year-old man is flown in and is the first to arrive.

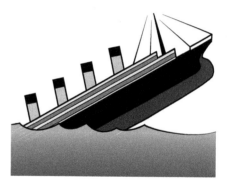

The patient is accompanied by his friend, Rose, and transferred to the resuscitation room. CPR is already taking place by the helicopter crew. A rectal temperature is 24°C, he has central cyanosis and no evidence of trauma.

i. How should a hypothermic patient be rewarded?

Heat loss should be prevented by removing the patient from the cold environment and removing wet clothing. **Passive re-warming** involves covering with warm blankets in a warm room and a warming rate of 0.5–2°C per hour can be expected. This is usually sufficient for mild hypothermia providing the patient can generate heat through shivering. **Active re-warming**, such as warm intravenous fluids and warmed oxygen, may achieve 1–2°C per hour of temperature rise and can be used for moderate hypothermia.

Severe hypothermia may require additional, more invasive methods, such as bladder irrigation, oesophageal warming tubes and peritoneal lavage, which may achieve 1–4°C per hour.

Extracorporeal methods, such as heated dialysis and cardiopulmonary bypass, may achieve a rate of 1–2°C per 5 minutes. This should be done wherever possible in a critical care setting. It has been shown that cardiopulmonary bypass is the most effective re-warming technique in severe hypothermia.

ii. What does this ECG show (Fig. 11.1)?

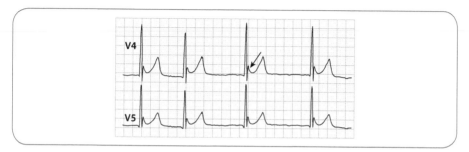

Figure 11.1.

There may be J waves on the ECG. These are characteristic, but not pathognomonic of hypothermia.

iii. When should CPR be stopped?

The lowest recorded survival temperature in a patient is 13.7°C, therefore although signs of cardiac and respiratory activity may appear absent, CPR should commence immediately and continue until further assessment can be made – 'you are not dead, until you are warm and dead.' All decisions to stop resuscitation should be taken as a team and with discussion with family members.

OUTCOME

Unfortunately, resuscitation attempts were unsuccessful despite active rewarming through peritoneal and pleural lavage. Following a long resuscitative effort CPR was discontinued once the temperature was normalized. The patient's partner was successfully treated with passive warming. She was referred to the psychiatrist as other passengers had reported that she was seen trying to jump off the ship prior to it hitting the iceberg. She led a long and unhappy life plagued by a feeling of guilt for not letting her partner board the life raft with her.

CASE 12

Phileus Fogg, an English gentleman, presents to your emergency department complaining of shortness of breath. He also complains of some pain on breathing in deeply but thinks he probably pulled a muscle with heavy lifting. He is normally fit and well with no systemic symptoms. He occasionally smokes a pipe. He also reports having recently got back from a 'round the world trip' that took him 80 days. This involved long periods of travelling in cramped conditions, including a long trip on a paddle steamer. On examination, his BP is 125/70, heart rate is 125 and regular and his oxygen saturations are 93% on air. He is afebrile and you notice that his left leg is swollen and

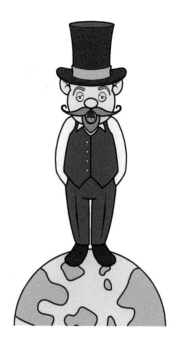

warm, but Mr Fogg says, 'don't worry about that, it is probably from a bite or something.' A chest radiograph is unremarkable and an ECG shows a sinus tachycardia.

i. What is the most likely diagnosis?

With the history of shortness of breath, pleuritic chest pain and leg swelling on a background of recent air travel and relative inactivity, a pulmonary embolism must be considered. This is a blockage in the pulmonary arterial system that usually results from a venous thrombosis, more commonly in the lower limb or pelvis. It can cause damage to the lung at the site of the thrombus and damage secondary to hypoxia to other organs.

ii. What is the Well's score?

The Well's score (Fig. 12.1) was devised to stratify the probability of a deep vein thrombosis (DVT) or pulmonary embolus (PE). For the diagnosis of a PE, the Well's score consists of the following:

A score of six points or more gives a high probability for a PE and a CTPA should be arranged. A score of two points or less gives a low probability of a PE.

Clinically a DVT is suspected	3 points
Alternative diagnosis is less likely than PE	3 points
Tachycardia (pulse >100)	1.5 points
Previous history of DVT or PE	1.5 points
Recent immobilization (>3 days) or surgery in the past 4 weeks	1.5 points
Malignancy or palliative patient	1 point
Haemoptysis	1 point

Figure 12.1.

iii. What is the most common ECG finding for this condition?

Although medical students and juniors are often taught that with a PE, a deep S wave in lead I, a Q wave in lead III and an inverted T wave in lead III (S1, Q3, T3) are the classic findings, the most common finding is in fact a sinus tachycardia. This is seen in 44% of patients. Other signs include right bundle branch block (18%), right axis deviation or right strain.

OUTCOME

A CTPA was performed, which confirmed the diagnosis of a PE, and the patient underwent treatment with subcutaneous low molecular weight heparin before being switched to a direct oral anticoagulant. Mr Fogg self-discharged stating that he needed to be back to his Gentleman's club by the end of the 80 days to collect his £20,000 wager.

CASE 13

The Swiss Robinson family turn up as a group to your GP surgery. They have just returned from the East Indies where they were shipwrecked on an island for several years. Fritz Robinson, the eldest son, is the focus of this consultation. He describes a rash over his foot. It was quite itchy and he thought maybe it was a bite or something. He is otherwise systemically well. The rash is shown (Fig. 13.1).

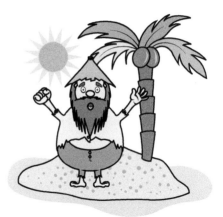

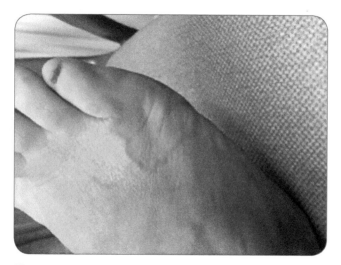

Figure 13.1.

i. What does this image show?

The image shows the track of a parasitic worm infection known as cutaneous larva migrans. It is sometimes known as the 'creeping eruption' and is a clinical diagnosis. It is caused by the accidental penetration of hookworm larvae through the skin. These larvae may be found in the soil or sand and then enter the human via broken skin or hair follicles. Their normal hosts are the intestines of animals such as dogs and cats, but in humans they are unable to penetrate the basement membrane. They therefore live and move around the epidermis, hence this type of rash. This means humans are known as an 'end host.'

ii. Where is this condition found?

Cutaneous larva migrans is one of the most common skin diseases in those returning from the tropics. Common areas include Asia, the Caribbean, Australia and Central and South America.

iii. What is the treatment for this condition?

Although this condition is self-limiting and, if left untreated, the larvae will simply die after a period of migrating around the epidermis, most people opt for treatment. Topical treatment can be applied but, if more widespread, an oral anthelmintic agent such as albendazole may be given. The rash can be intensely itchy and so adjunct therapies such as an antihistamine may also be used.

OUTCOME

Fritz was given a course of albendazole and his itching improved within 24–48 hours. His lesion slowly resolved over the course of 1–2 weeks. He was referred to counselling as he found adjusting to urban life difficult following his stay on the island and later turned to alcohol for solace.

CASE 14

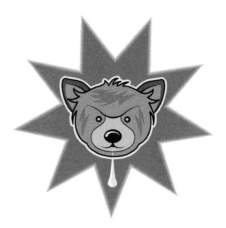

You are asked to see a patient who has been brought in by ambulance to the emergency department. You understand he is from Tasmania and that his family were concerned that the patient woke up this morning with one side of his face appearing to be drooping and he was salivating on that side. He also was finding it frustrating as he was unable to get his words out. This was making him more annoyed. He is not a smoker but his family report he is always fairly stressed out and he is a diabetic. On examination he has marked facial droop, expressive dysphasia and some subtle right-sided weakness, and you note that he is in atrial fibrillation.

i. Is this patient a candidate for thrombolysis?

No. The clinical picture suggests this patient has had a stroke. The current guidelines state that if patients have had an ischaemic stroke, then thrombolysis can be considered within 3 hours. This has been extended to 4.5 hours and studies are looking at even longer. There are strict criteria and contraindications and in this case, the patient woke up with his symptoms. This means that it is not possible to determine the exact onset of symptoms. Once they have been initially assessed, using an ABC approach, a potential thrombolysis candidate needs a CT scan to exclude haemorrhage, which would obviously be a contraindication.

You are asked to see the Tasmanian patient because he has developed a fever and has an increased respiratory rate. Nursing staff tell you that shortly prior to coming onto their shift, he ate everything he could get his hands on. On examination his oxygen saturations are 94% on 4 litres, he has crackles on his right base and he is febrile and tachycardic.

ii. What is the most likely diagnosis?

It is likely this patient has aspirated. This is a common and potentially life-threatening complication and stroke patients should be promptly assessed by a Speech and Language therapist to ensure a safe swallow.

iii. What is the CHADS2VAC score?

It is a score that aims to predict the risk of stroke or thromboembolism in patients with atrial fibrillation (Fig. 14.1). In female patients with a score of two or more and male patients with a score of one or more, anticoagulation medication is recommended.

Score for stroke risk in patients with atrial fibrillation (CHA, DS, VASc)	
Congestive heart failure	1 point
Hypertension	1 point
Age ≥75 years	2 points
Age 65 and 74 years	1 point
Diabetes	1 point
Stroke/TIA/thromboembolism	2 points
Vascular disease	1 point
Female	1 point

Figure 14.1.

OUTCOME

The Tasmanian patient initially deteriorated and went to ICU. However, he responded well to antibiotics and was taken off the ventilator. His enthusiasm and motivation meant his rehab progressed swiftly, although he never fully regained his speech. He was discharged home with carers for support but his voracious appetite put a huge strain on the meals on wheels service.

CASE 15

Your next patient in your busy GP morning clinic arrives. He introduces himself as Hercules and you are immediately impressed with his size and stature. He reports some heavy lifting over the past few months. Yesterday, this 25 year old lifted a large boulder and developed severe pain in his back. He denies any bladder or bowel disturbances. A full neurological examination is performed, which is normal, and he has some pain on straight leg raise.

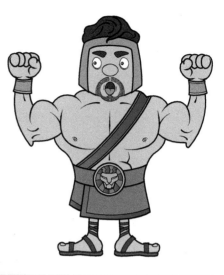

i. What are red flag features for back pain?

These are features that suggest there may be a more sinister underlying cause for the back pain, including discitis, malignancy or cauda equina (Fig. 15.1).

Age <16 or >50	History of malignancy
Unexplained weight loss	Fevers or rigors
Long-term steroid use	Saddle anaesthesia and reduced anal tone
Urinary retention	Erectile dysfunction

Figure 15.1.

ii. What would be a reasonable pain regime for this patient?

Pain relief is the mainstay of treatment together with early mobilization. Early mobilization can only be achieved if there is adequate pain relief and so an aggressive regime should be adopted. Back pain is a leading cause of time off work in the UK and costs the country millions of pounds. It is important to warn patients that they may be debilitated for some time. Pain management should follow an increasing strength stepwise approach but would start with an NSAID, tramadol (or codeine) and a short course of diazepam if the pain is really bad to help relieve muscle spasms. (Note: there is some recent evidence that finds no overall benefit with paracetamol for back pain.) Neuropathic agents such as amitriptyline or gabapentin could be considered if there is sciatica or nerve root pain.

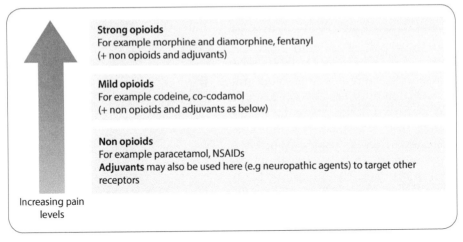

Strong opioids
For example morphine and diamorphine, fentanyl
(+ non opioids and adjuvants)

Mild opioids
For example codeine, co-codamol
(+ non opioids and adjuvants as below)

Non opioids
For example paracetamol, NSAIDs
Adjuvants may also be used here (e.g neuropathic agents) to target other
receptors

Increasing pain
levels

Figure 15.2.

It is worth noting that the World Health Organization pain ladder (Fig. 15.2) was created for cancer pain relief, although it is more widely used in the management of chronic pain due to other causes.

iii. What is cauda equina syndrome?

This is a neurological emergency, normally managed by the orthopaedic team in close consultation with their spinal surgical colleagues, depending on a hospital's policy. Damage to the cauda equina causes lower motor neurone signs; causes include trauma or compression (from a herniated disc, bleeding, malignancy, infection or fractures). Any patient with saddle anaesthesia or altered sensation when wiping from toileting, urinary retention or dribbling, incomplete erections and decreased sphincter tone on a rectal examination in the context of severe back pain should have an urgent orthopaedic opinion. Imaging would include an urgent MRI and surgical decompression may be warranted.

OUTCOME

Hercules was discharged home with good analgesia. Unfortunately, due to his increasing number of days off work, his brother Hades took over his business and Hercules is currently in an employment tribunal citing unfair dismissal.

CASE 16

This patient was referred to your surgical take and brought in by his loyal
canine friend in the early hours of the
morning complaining of right upper
quadrant pain. His friend was asked by
the matron to wait outside due to the
strict no dogs (except guide dogs) policy in the hospital. The pain is constant
in nature and he has vomited once. He
also feels very feverish. He is normally
well, although he describes having
pains on that side for several months,

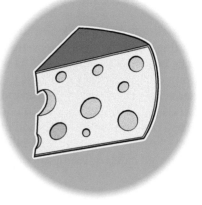

worse after a meal. He reports that the past few days he has been enjoying a
'particularly good Wensleydale.' On examination he is febrile at 38°C, looks
flushed, with a heart rate of 105, BP 120/70 and RR of 15. His saturations are
100%. He is Murphy's positive and the rest of his abdomen is soft. A rectal
examination is unremarkable. His bloods show a markedly raised CRP and
white cell count, with normal LFTs and a normal amylase. An erect chest radiograph does not show any free air.

i. What is the most likely diagnosis?

The most likely diagnosis is cholecystytis. However, other possible causes of
abdominal pain must be considered including hepatitis, pancreatitis, pyelone-
phritis and appendicitis.

ii. How would you manage this patient?

As always, an ABC focused approach should be adopted. Blood cultures should
be taken, ideally before commencing antibiotics, which should include anaerobic and gram-negative cover. Pain relief is also important and patients should
initially be on free fluids before introducing a low fat diet in consultation with
the dieticians. Patients will be offered a laparoscopic cholecystectomy. Ideally
this would be done within 48 hours, but due to operating list logistics, this is
often not possible. Therefore, patients are often brought back as an elective
admission after a few weeks when the inflammation has settled, as otherwise
this can make the operation technically more difficult.

Biliary colic is pain in the absence of infection due to gallstones. This is most
likely the pain this patient was suffering from previously.

iii. What are the signs on ultrasound that would support this diagnosis?

This question is often asked in exams and by surgeons on ward rounds. The findings include pericholecystic fluid, gallbladder wall thickening, the presence of stones or sludge and Murphy's sign at ultrasound. This is where the point of maximal tenderness is in the right upper quadrant when the gallbladder is seen on ultrasound. Clinically, Murphy's sign is elicited by placing your hands in the midclavicular line just below the ribs and asking the patient to take a deep breath in. As the gallbladder comes in close contact with the examiner's fingers, the patient will either wince or catch their breath. Absence of this on the left side while present on the right makes this a positive Murphy's sign.

OUTCOME

The patient was found to have lots of gallstones on ultrasound. He was booked in for an elective cholecystectomy. He missed his operation as he was said to be in a meeting with Richard Branston to try and get him to land on the moon to see if he really was made of cheese.

CASE 17

An elderly gentleman in a long grey cloak is wheeled into the emergency department. He tells you he is many hundred years old and fell off a white horse onto his left side. He knows he should not be horse riding at his age but tells you it was vital he joined his hairy footed friends on an important quest to return some jewellery. He has pain in the left groin and cannot walk. His left leg appears shorter than the right and the foot is turned outwards. You obtain a radiograph of the hips (Fig. 17.1).

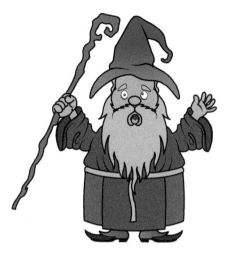

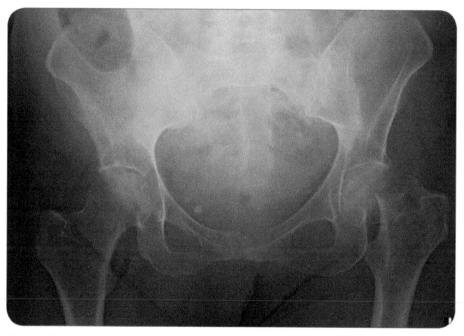

Figure 17.1.

i. What is the diagnosis?

The radiograph demonstrates a left intracapsular neck of femur fracture.

ii. What are the treatment options, and what is the anatomical basis for this?

This can be treated with reduction of the fracture and internal fixation with cannulated screws in young patients or non-displaced fractures. Displaced fractures in the elderly should be treated with hemiarthroplasty or total hip replacement. The blood supply of the femoral head in adults is mainly via retinacular vessels along the femoral neck and intramedullary vessels. This blood supply is disrupted in displaced fractures, leading to a high risk of avascular necrosis, making replacement, rather than fixation, a sensible option.

iii. What can be done to prevent further fractures?

Neck of femur fractures are a type of fragility fracture indicating that the patient is likely to have osteoporosis. Other fragility fractures include Colles wrist fractures and vertebral body wedge fractures. There should be assessment and treatment of osteoporosis, which may include calcium and vitamin D supplementation and bisphosphonate therapy.

OUTCOME

The patient was transferred to a community hospital where he began mobilizing with the aid of a stick, which he quickly discarded as he preferred using a staff. He was delighted with the outcome of his hip replacement and continued to enjoy long journeys with his crew of friends.

CASE 18

A very tall, friendly man stumbles into the emergency department with a young child and carrying what looks to be a large, long trumpet. He drinks from a strange substance from a bottle and has loud flatulence, causing other patients to stare. He tells you his hands and face are growing and he has had to buy a new, bigger hat. He has also started bumping into

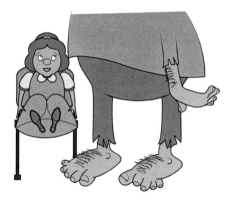

things due to bad eyesight. On examination he does have large spade-like hands, coarse facial features and his peripheral visual fields are affected on both eyes.

i. What is the likely diagnosis?

The diagnosis of acromegaly should be considered. This is due to a growth hormone-secreting pituitary tumour.

ii. How does this diagnosis explain the visual loss?

A bitemporal hemianopia is caused by compression of the optic chiasm by an enlarging pituitary mass. As fibres cross over the temporal field of each eye is affected.

The diagram shown (**Fig. 18.1**) is worth remembering as it helps to explain all visual field losses and the causes of them. For instance, a lesion of the optic tract on the right will result in a left homonymous hemianopia.

iii. What are the treatment options?

Treatment can be medical or surgical to prevent further growth hormone release. This can be achieved medically by using somatostatin analogues such as ocreotide or dopamine agonists such as bromocryptine. Surgical removal of the tumour can be achieved via a trans-sphenoidal approach.

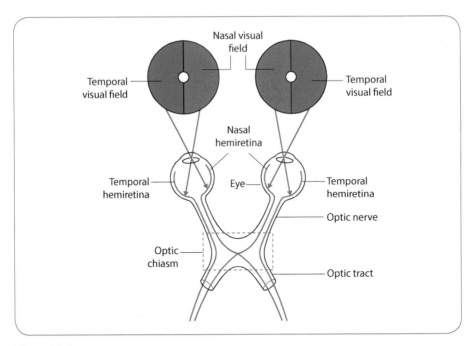

Figure 18.1.

The patient went away to consider his diagnosis and treatment options. He reported getting frequent nightmares regarding surgery. Finally he decided that he quite liked being very big and that he did not want any treatment at all.

CASE 19

A young orphan is brought by a carer to the emergency department with a painful right leg. He looks hungry and malnourished and after scoffing down a sandwich askes you 'please sir can I have some more?' He lets you examine him. He has bruises all over his chest and arms and a very painful swollen leg. His carers are unsure how long he has been like this and do not remember any injury. The carers are quite evasive and want you to give the all clear quickly and become a bit annoyed when you say you need to do some tests. You obtain a radiograph of the pelvis and legs (Fig. 19.1).

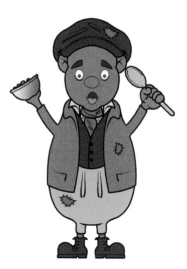

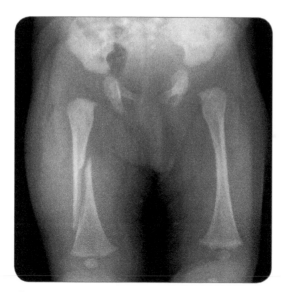

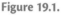

Figure 19.1.

i. What are the concerns regarding this injury?

This is a spiral fracture of the femur in a young child. Spiral fractures indicate a twisting force such as a pull by a careless parent and should raise suspicion, especially in a non-ambulatory child. The possibility of non-accidental injury (NAI) should be carefully considered.

ii. What factors may make you suspicious of NAI?

NAI is unfortunately not uncommon and there have been several notable cases recently. Healthcare professionals have a duty to recognize and protect vulnerable children. Delay in seeking help, inconsistent history or incompatibility with mechanism of injury, multiple injuries and abnormal interaction with parents should all raise a suspicion of a NAI. A full examination should be performed and other injuries should be actively sought by trained professionals and further investigation by the paediatric team if any concerns are present.

iii. What investigations are ordered if there is a concern of NAI?

If a significant concern is present, the child should undergo a comprehensive clinical examination. A skeletal survey can be performed to look for any fractures (especially ribs), a CT head scan to look for intracranial haemorrhage (from shaken baby) and fundoscopy performed to look for retinal haemorrhages.

OUTCOME

A safeguarding alert was made regarding the patient. While on the ward the patient had a few unsavoury visitors and there were reports of watches and wallets going missing. He was later put into a foster home where he thrived.

CASE 20

A 45-year-old sailor comes into your GP practice with a painful left toe. The receptionist informs you that she has had to tell him to extinguish his pipe several times and you make a note to refer him to the smoking cessation service. He reports a several hour history of a red, painful and swollen toe. He denies any trauma to it and does not feel feverish. On lifestyle questioning he reports a diet consisting mainly of spinach and he drinks upwards of

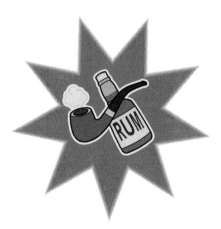

20 units per week of rum. On examination the metatarsophalangeal joint of the left toe is red, hot, shiny and inflamed. You suspect gout.

i. What is gout?

Gout is a form of arthritis that is caused by increased levels of uric acid. These increased levels can either be caused by reduced filtration by the kidneys or by producing too much uric acid. This leads to the deposition of crystals in the joints, which causes the symptoms. Diet plays a role with an increased risk of gout in patients who consume high levels of alcohol, meat and seafood. Obesity is also a risk factor. Interestingly, studies have shown that foods rich in purine, such as spinach, peas and lentils, do not in fact cause a raised uric acid. Issues with excretion, such as kidney failure, also can cause gout. Psoriasis and diuretic and aspirin use are also risk factors.

ii. What does microscopy show?

This is for some reason a common examination question. Following joint aspiration, the synovial fluid is used for polarized light microscopy. This will show needle-shaped crystals with negative birefringence (as opposed to **pseudogout**, which will be rhomboid in shape and show **positive** birefringence) (Fig. 20.1). Joint aspiration may also help in excluding a diagnosis of septic arthritis.

iii. What is the treatment for gout?

The treatment for gout can be split into symptomatic and prevention measures. Immediate treatment involves pain relief. NSAIDs are used first line but are used with caution in some instances and a proton pump inhibitor may be concurrently prescribed to protect the gastrointestinal tract. Colchichine can be used if NSAIDs are contraindicated at a dose of 500 micrograms 2–4 times a day, increased until adequate pain relief is achieved or the side effects of

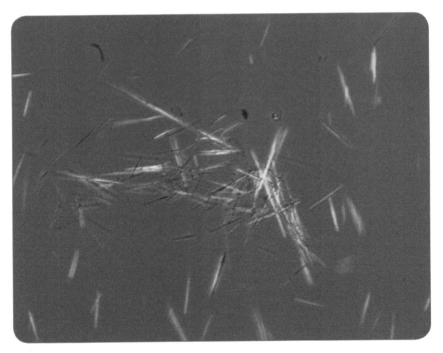

Figure 20.1.

diarrhoea become problematic, whichever is first (up to a maximum total dose of 6 mg). Steroids can also be used to treat gout.

Allopurinol, a xanthine oxidase inhibitor is used in the prevention of gout. This prevents the breakdown of xanthine to uric acid. It is not prescribed during an acute attack as this may worsen symptoms. Lifestyle measures such as increased exercise, weight loss and reduced alcohol consumption should also be employed.

OUTCOME

Following a course of NSAIDs, the patient's toe improves. However, he returns having been in a drunken fight with a larger man over a lady. Having cut back on his spinach consumption he is easily outmuscled and re-attends with multiple injuries. After tending to these he is referred to the drug and alcohol team.

CASE 21

The Easter Bunny comes into the GP clinic. He was recently diagnosed with type 2 diabetes and wanted to try and alter his diet in an attempt to control his blood sugar levels. He reports finding this very hard as he finds the temptation of Easter eggs too much to resist. His blood glucose levels are consistently around 17 mmol/L. You decide to prescribe metformin.

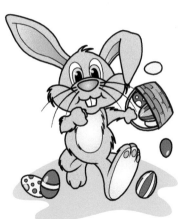

i. What is the action of metformin?

Metformin is a biguanide and works by decreasing gluconeogenesis in the liver. It also increases the peripheral sensitivity of insulin. It can only work in the presence of endogenous insulin and so there must be some functioning pancreatic islet cells available in the body for it to work.

ii. What are the side effects of metformin?

Metformin is generally well tolerated, with gastrointestinal disturbances being the most common side effect. However, an important caution that is a favourite in exams is its potential to cause a lactic acidosis. Therefore, any patient with renal impairment should be monitored closely and if severe, alternative therapies considered. At times of a sudden decrease in renal function or hypoxia, such as during sepsis, metformin should be halted and reviewed at a later date. This is an important initial task of an admitting house officer to do, as it can always be restarted later.

iii. How often should a patient with type 2 diabetes have an eye test?

Annual screening is recommended for patients with diabetes. There are a number of significant eye problems associated with poor glucose control and it is worth reading around this subject, as the different stages are often mentioned in exam questions.

OUTCOME

The Easter Bunny was started on metformin. He altered his diet and began delivering real eggs instead of the chocolate kind. This caused uproar amongst the local schoolchildren and he was forced to resign his job and move to the countryside.

CASE 22

A 45-year-old well-dressed gentle-man presents to your GP clinic. He says he works for the Government and that he has come to see you as he is worried about his lifestyle. He says his secretary recommended coming to see you as she reports he is drinking too much. He says he mainly drinks martinis and that this equals approximately 30 units per week. He describes several flings with women from abroad and that he is often getting into fights. He also is concerned he is getting too old for his job and is wondering if you can complete a sick note for him for a few days following a recent incident where he jumped off a moving train.

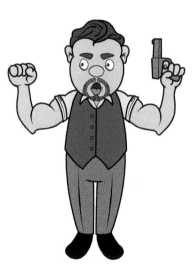

i. What is the CAGE questionnaire and what is it used for?

The CAGE questionnaire can be a useful screening tool for alcohol dependence. It consists of four questions and uses the pneumonic CAGE:

a) Have you ever felt that you should **C**ut down your drinking?
b) Has anyone **A**nnoyed you by criticizing your drinking habits?
c) Have you ever felt **G**uilty or bad about your drinking?
d) Have you ever had an **E**yeopener in the morning (a drink to get you going, calm you down or get rid of a hangover in the morning)?

A score of 2 or more indicates a high index of suspicion and scoring 4 is diagnostic for alcoholism.

ii. What is the weekly recommended intake for males and females?

The current recommendations are that both men and women should not exceed 14 units per week of alcohol. If this maximum number is consumed, it should be spread out over more than 3 days, not consumed in one session. Binge drinking is harmful to health.

In pregnancy, alcohol should be avoided for the first 3 months as it may increase the risk of miscarriage. If patients decide to drink, they should consume no more than 1–2 units once or twice a week. This is because there is no evidence that there is harm to a baby at these levels; however, the more you drink, the greater the risk of complications to the baby. The Chief Medical Officer advises avoiding alcohol all together in pregnancy in the most recent guidelines.

iii. How long can patients self-certify, and what is a Med3 form?

Patients can claim Statutory Sick Pay for any illness of 7 calendar days or less by self-certifying and completing a form. In the past there were several types of sickness certificate but these have been replaced by one Statement of Fitness For Work. The initial certificate can last up to 3 months. In complex cases, you can recommend an occupational health assessment. A copy of the sick note issued to this gentleman is shown (Fig. 22.1). Under the Official Secrets Act 1989, MI5 insisted we blank out his name and address and date of birth.

Statement of Fitness for Work
For social security or Statutory Sick Pay

Patient's name	Mr, Mrs, Miss, Ms
I assessed your case on:	❶ 15 / 12 / 2018
and, because of the following condition(s):	❷ Multiple injuries Anxiety and depression

I advise you that:
❸ ☐ you are not fit for work.
❹ ☒ you may be fit for work taking account of the following advice:

If available, and with your employer's agreement, you may benefit from:

☐ a phased return to work   ☒ amended duties
❺
☐ altered hours   ☐ workplace adaptations

Comments, including functional effects of your condition(s):
❻
avoid heavy lifting (over 5kg), heavy drinking
and driving motorised vehicles over rooftops

This will be the case for	❼
or from	❽ 15 / 12 / 2018 to 15 / 02 / 2019

❾ I will/will not need to assess your fitness for work again at the end of this period.
(Please delete as applicable)

Doctor's signature	E Schwarz
Date of statement	15 / 12 / 2018
Doctor's address	Stars Consulting Rooms Hollywood Los Angeles

Unique ID: Med 3 04/10

Figure 22.1.

OUTCOME

The patient engaged with local drug and alcohol services and re-commenced active service. Following his return from a subsequent assignment, he represented with a virulent urethral discharge and was referred to the local genitourinary clinic.

CASE 23

A fireman is rushed to the emergency department having been brought directly from a house fire in a small Welsh village where he was found unconscious in a burning room. He is alert and able to talk with a croaky voice and tells you his name is Sam. He has extensive burns across his body. You note some singeing of his nasal hairs and burns on his face.

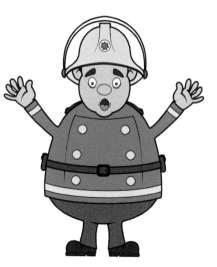

i. What are the signs of an inhalational injury, and what is the significance of this?

Inhalational or airway burns are suggested by singeing of the nasal hair/beard or soot around the mouth. Other clues may be facial burns, a patient with a hoarse voice, wheezy chest or cough as well as burns sustained in an enclosed space. Any of these should raise the suspicion of a possible airway issue and an anaesthetist should be involved early to consider early intubation before further swelling makes this more difficult.

ii. How are burns classified and measured?

There are several ways to classify burns but the widely known 'degree classification' (first-degree, second-degree, etc) has become obsolete. Instead, burns are classified into four categories by the depth of the burn:

a) **Superficial** – affect the epidermis only and cause erythema.
b) **Superficial partial thickness** – painful burns which cause blistering and remain sensate (i.e. they are usually very painful).
c) **Deep dermal** – reduced sensation and capillary refill time.
d) **Full-thickness burns** – are leathery, do not blanch and are insensate.

Burns can be measured by percentage body area involved, which can be estimated using the Wallace Rule of Nine (**Fig. 23.1**) or, more accurately, using a Lund and Browder chart.

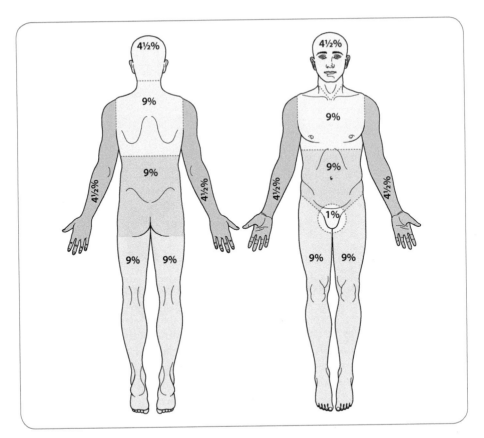

Figure 23.1.

iii. When do patients require fluid resuscitation, and how is this calculated?

Fluid resuscitation is required in burns of more than 15–20% of the total body surface area (TBSA). Requirements can be estimated using the Parkland formula of 3–4 mL/kg/TBSA(%), with half of this given over the first 8 hours post burn and the remaining fluid given over the next 16 hours, with Hartmann's solution being the preferred crystalloid.

OUTCOME

The Fireman was intubated due to suspected airway risk and fluid resuscitated due to his 50% mixed depth burns. Despite best care in the local burns centre he unfortunately passed away. The dog he had entered the burning building to rescue lived a long and happy life.

CASE 24

A 5-year-old boy is brought into the department by his father with bleeding from his right nostril. He is slightly wooden in appearance but he assures you he is a real boy. You check his observations and note that he is haemodynamically stable with no tachycardia or hypotension. You examine his elongated nose to look for a bleeding point.

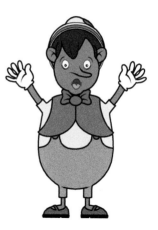

i. Where is the most likely location of a bleeding point?

Ninety percent of bleeding points are situated anteriorly, originating from the Little's area (a vascular bundle) on the nasal septum. This area can be compressed by pinching the nose, which should be tried as an initial first aid for a period of at least 10 minutes. Cold compressions, for example frozen peas, can be placed on the back of the neck and this can also aid in stemming the flow. Posterior epistaxis is far less common and more difficult to control.

ii. What are the precipitating causes?

Epistaxis is often caused by local irritation or trauma. Other risk factors include hypertension, coagulation abnormalities and taking anticoagulant medications such as warfarin, especially if this is not well controlled.

iii. What are the management options?

If the bleeding is not controlled by first aid measures, other options include cauterization of an obvious bleeding point or nasal packing with balloon nasal packs or ribbon gauze. If these fail to control bleeding, an ENT surgeon may consider ligation of contributory blood vessels.

OUTCOME

The bleeding was controlled by anterior nasal packing and later cauterization of the bleeding point by an ENT surgeon. Unfortunately, due to an ongoing uncontrolled nasal growth the bleeding recurred, requiring ligation of the external carotid artery.

CASE 25

A 33-year-old gentleman presents to the emergency department with a painful finger. He had been using a bow and arrow with his band of merry men when suddenly he felt a snap and had immediate pain in his finger. When you examine him his index finger is held straight and he is unable to flex at the distal interphalangeal joint.

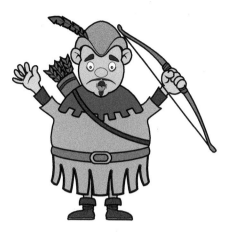

i. What is the most likely diagnosis?

He most likely has an avulsion of the flexor digitorum profundus (FDP) tendon from the base of the distal phalanx. This is normally caused by eccentric contraction of the flexor tendon and is commonly referred to as a 'jersey finger.'

ii. Would a radiograph be of help here?

Yes. The injury can be a rupture of the tendon itself or avulsion of a bony fragment. Radiographs will not show tendinous lesions but may show a bony avulsion fragment. This fragment often stops the tendon retracting to the palm and can be fixed back to the distal phalanx, whereas tendon avulsions require repair.

iii. Can you explain the anatomy of the flexor tendons of the fingers, and how they are tested?

The digits are flexed by two muscle tendons. The flexor digitorum superficialis (FDS) muscle lies superficially in the forearm and its tendons split to insert on to the middle phalanx of each finger, causing flexion at the proximal interphalangeal joints. FDP tendon lies deeper in the forearm and causes flexion at the distal interphalangeal joint (DIPJ). To do this it must pass through the split FDS tendon. FDS is tested by holding all the other digits straight and asking the patient to flex the finger. FDP is tested by holding the remainder of the finger straight and asking the patient to flex the DIPJ (Figs. 25.1a, b).

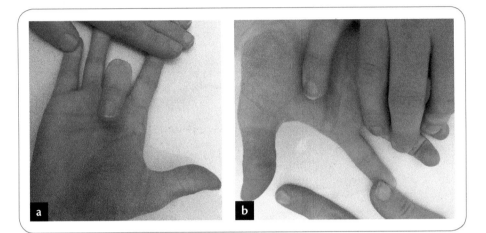

Figures 25.1a, b.

Robin underwent direct repair of the FDP tendon by a hand surgeon and was back stealing from the rich and giving to the poor within 8 weeks. A snap general election was held, for which he stood as leader of his party of merry men. Despite this his socialist ideals never caught on and he was branded an outcast.

CASE 26

An evil astronaut presented to the GP with a few month history of dysphagia and weight loss. He felt like food was getting stuck in his throat on swallowing. He is an ex heavy smoker and his only other medical history to note is that he suffered severe burns to his lower limbs as a young adult, requiring extensive grafting. Although the room is well lit, he prefers to sit on the dark side.

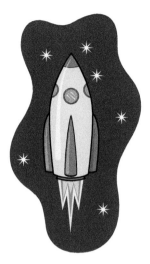

On examination he has a marked inspiratory stridor but is able to talk in complete sentences. His oxygen saturations are 98% on air.

i. What would be a differential diagnosis for this man's stridor?

Stridor is a loud, harsh pitched sound that usually is heard on inspiration but may also occur on expiration (or sometimes both). It indicates some narrowing of the respiratory system and is caused by turbulent flow. Stridor is a sign that should be taken very seriously and it is important that these patients are prioritized in an emergency department. Separating acute from chronic stridor is important, as more often acute stridor is more life threatening. Stridor can be caused by many conditions but a differential would include:

- Something intrinsic (e.g. a foreign body or food bolus, oedema from anaphylaxis, trauma or inhalation injury).
- Something extrinsic (e.g. tumour such as a squamous cell carcinoma of the larynx, oesophagus or trachea).
- Infection such as epiglottitis, severe laryngitis or retropharyngeal abscess.

Remember that in children the causes also include croup, epiglottitis, anaphylaxis and inhaled foreign bodies.

ii. What imaging would be arranged?

Initial imaging would include plain radiographs of the neck, contrast studies or CT and also direct visualization by an ENT doctor.

iii. How would you manage a patient with stridor?

As always, an ABCDE approach should be used and this patient will most likely have a problem with their airway. Initial management includes giving oxygen and suctioning if anything was visualized and back blows if an inhaled object is suspected. Should this patient deteriorate, anaesthetic support will be needed and the patient may need to be intubated or have an urgent cricothyroidotomy or tracheostomy.

OUTCOME

The patient was diagnosed with oesophageal cancer, likely secondary to his heavy smoking. He was last seen on a Jeremy Kyle show titled, 'I am your father. Lie detector tests'.

CASE 27

You see your next patient, a 32-year-old bear, in a busy emergency department. He is rushed through to the resus department with his oldest faithful friend. He was searching in the forest for his favourite food – honey – when he came across a hive. Unable to control his insatiable appetite, he put his hand into a hive and was stung several times. He then became very short of breath and wheezy with lip swelling. By the time the paramedics arrived, his airway was becoming compromised and he was unable to complete sentences. His friend was a first aider and had placed him in the recovery position. His friend was very agitated, jumping up and down nearby. On examination in the department, his saturations are 92%, his heart rate is 125 and his BP is 98/40. He has marked facial oedema and lip swelling and you note marked stridor.

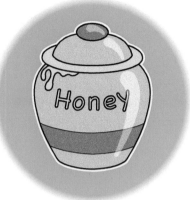

i. Given the likely diagnosis, what is the immediate treatment?

As always, you should assess an unwell patient using the ABCDE rule. In this case, the patient is suffering from anaphylaxis from a bee sting. Such patients are shocked (hypotensive, tachycardic and tachypnoeic) and are in peri-arrest. Therefore, immediate treatment is with intramuscular adrenaline. This should have already been given by the paramedics and is one of the few drugs that it is essential to know the doses of, as it is time dependent and patients respond quickly. For anaphylaxis, the adult dose is 500 µg (0.5 mL) of 1 in 1,000 adrenaline intramuscularly.

ii. What is the treatment dose for a child?

This is again a very useful dose to remember, hence its inclusion, and is based on 10 µg/kg to a maximum of 500 µg. It is useful to just remember that a child aged 6–12 years should be given 300 µg (0.3 mL) and a child under 6 years 150 µg (0.15 mL).

iii. Given the diagnosis, what other advice/treatment should be given to the patient?

This patient should be advised to avoid the precipitant, in this case bees. He should carry an autoinjector (Epipen®) that should be in date and a medic alert bracelet to inform responders of his condition.

OUTCOME

The patient responded to the adrenaline, although he required several doses. He was also given steroid and an antihistamine as he developed a widespread urticarial rash. He was observed overnight as a precaution and discharged in the morning. Despite advice, he could not abstain from honey, although he was pleased to find out he could obtain it in jars from his local supermarket. He continued to snack throughout the day, requiring a referral to the dieticians.

CASE 28

A 72 year old presented to the emergency department having collapsed in his garden. He is accompanied by his lawyer and his son and lots of godchildren. Three other men wearing long coats and dark glasses initially accompanied the patient, although they left quickly to 'settle some unfinished business.' The only person who witnessed the collapse was his 4-year-old grandson, who saw him clutch his chest prior to the collapse. An ECG (Fig. 28.1) was taken in the emergency department.

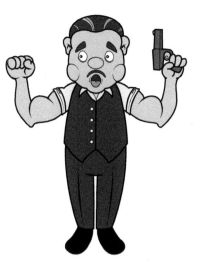

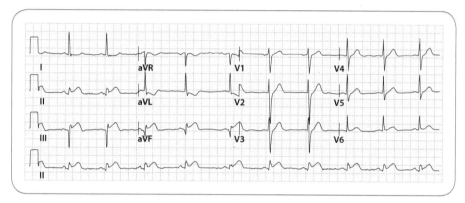

Figure 28.1.

i. What does this ECG show?

The ECG demonstrates a sinus rhythm, with a rate of approximately 65. There is no axis deviation. There is ST elevation in leads II, III and aVF (inferior leads) and ST depression in leads I and aVL (lateral leads). ST elevation of more than 1 mm in two or more consecutive chest leads or 2 mm in two or more limb leads is diagnostic of an ST elevation myocardial infarction.

ii. Where is the likely lesion?

The ECG findings would correspond with a lesion in the right coronary artery. The ECG overleaf (Fig. 28.2) shows the different leads, their vascular supply and the region of the heart.

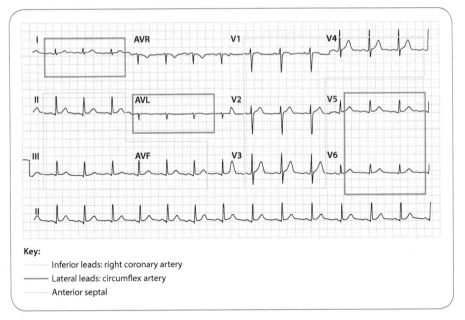

Key:

-------- Inferior leads: right coronary artery

———— Lateral leads: circumflex artery

-------- Anterior septal

Figure 28.2.

iii. What is the management of this patient?

As always, an ABCDE approach should be taken to the patient. This patient needs urgent percutaneous coronary intervention or, if not available in your hospital, thrombolysis. 'Time is muscle' and so this should be organized urgently. In most centres, ambulances have the facility to fax across ECGs straight to the coronary care unit to alert the team in advance.

OUTCOME

Unfortunately, despite the paramedic and emergency physician's best efforts, the patient had a cardiac arrest and died. The attending physician mysteriously died in a car accident in which he was found in the boot. No arrests were made.

CASE 29

A patient is seen in your GP clinic requesting a repeat prescription of nasal decongestants. You note six of his friends are waiting patiently in the waiting room with a variety of garden tools. One is asleep and one appears very cross at having to wait for so long. You perform a perfect consultation, using a tried and tested consultation model and as you are about to show him out of your clinic, he stops you and tells you he is about to start a family with his new wife. You notice that he is of short stature with a large head and prominent forehead. You remember that his wife is of normal stature and is normally well except having recently suffered from a nasty case of narcolepsy.

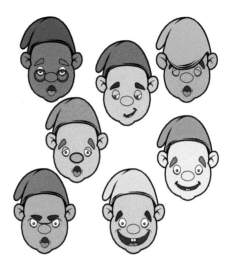

i. What are the chances of this patient's offspring having achondroplasia?

Achondroplasia is inherited in an autosomal dominant fashion. This means that only a single copy of the abnormal gene is necessary to express the disease in offspring. The risk of passing this down to their child is therefore 50% with **each** pregnancy. If two people with achondroplasia have a child together, there is a 25% chance of having an unaffected child, a 50% chance of having a child with achondroplasia and a 25% chance of having a child with both dominant genes. In this latter case, the presence of both genes often leads to a premature death within the first few months of life (**Fig. 29.1**).

In this case, where only one parent is affected, the offspring have a 50% chance of having achondroplasia and a 50% chance of being unaffected. Subsequent offspring will also have the same subsequent risk as the probability is independent of previous pregnancies.

It should be remembered that 80% of new cases are due to a sporadic mutation, with normal stature parents.

ii. What are the characteristic features of achondroplasia?

Achondroplasia is a disproportionate dwarfism where the limbs are short compared with a normal sized trunk. Other classic features include large head with frontal bossing, flattened nasal bridge, bowed legs and trident hands. Intelligence is normal.

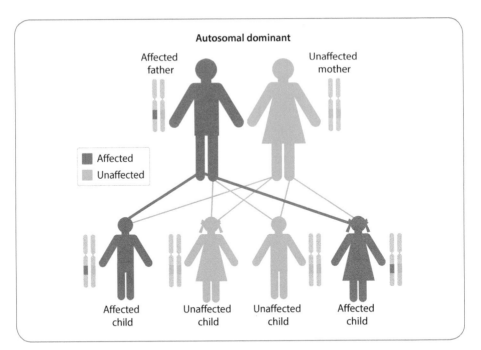

Autosomal dominant

Affected father — Unaffected mother

- ■ Affected
- □ Unaffected

Affected child — Unaffected child — Unaffected child — Affected child

Figure 29.1.

iii. What are the other modes of inheritance?

They can be autosomal dominant or recessive, meaning that the affected gene is located on any chromosome other than the sex chromosomes (X or Y). They can also be sex linked dominant or recessive, which are both more likely to affect males as they only have one X chromosome. Mitochondrial disorders are passed through mitochondrial DNA, which is always inherited from the mother. They can also be complex, meaning that there is an interaction of multiple genes or environmental factors.

OUTCOME

The wife became pregnant and gave birth to an achondroplasic child. Your patient became increasingly grumpy at his suspicions that he was not the father. He fell out with one of his happier colleagues, who always had a cheeky grin on his face, thinking that he may be responsible.

CASE 30

A Pacific blue tang fish comes into your clinic today. She is brought in by her friend, who is clowning around. Her friend is concerned that she is losing her memory. He has noticed

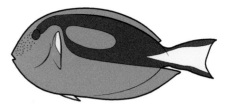

over the past 3 years that she keeps forgetting where she puts things and her short-term memory seems poor. She cannot remember where her family are and even forgot she could read. She speaks a variety of different dialects, including whale. She cannot remember if there is a family history of forgetfulness. Looking through her notes she does not have any medical conditions and just takes the occasional paracetamol. Her observations and clinical examination are normal and you suspect this patient may have signs of dementia.

i. What is the difference between dementia and delirium?

Dementia is a term used to describe a largely irreversible, progressive deterioration in cognition, memory, behaviour and personality without impairment of consciousness. Delirium describes a transient, acute and reversible impairment to mental state. It is also referred to as acute confusional state. The causes of delirium are wide ranging. Infection, constipation, pain and electrolyte disturbances are some of the most commonest causes on a care of the elderly ward.

ii. What are the possible treatable causes of dementia?

Although the commonest causes of dementia include Alzheimer's (slow progressive decline in cognition and impaired function) and vascular dementia (generalized small vessel disease or multiple infarcts, often more sudden and deterioration can be marked with each new infarct), there are some causes that need to be considered as they are potentially reversible/ differ in treatment. The triad of incontinence, gait disturbance and dementia, for example, should raise the suspicion of normal pressure hydrocephalus. This could be treated with a shunt (if the patient is a surgical candidate). Other abnormalities such as space-occupying lesions, hypothyroidism, vitamin B_{12} deficiency and Wilson's disease (and syphylis) should be considered.

iii. What does the DVLA advise with regards to driving?

Patients by law have to inform the DVLA with regards to driving and dementia. The DVLA will then decide whether further investigations are required and the patient may need to reapply on a yearly basis. If you as a doctor are aware that your patient is driving despite you telling them it is not allowed, it is your duty to inform the DVLA.

OUTCOME

The patient was referred to the memory clinic; however, after repeat missed appointments due to her forgetting the clinic time, she was not offered a further slot. She was last seen heading into the blue towards Sydney and social services believe she is a vulnerable adult.

CASE 31

RC is a 40-year-old man who presents to your GP outreach clinic with two lesions on his scalp (Figs. 31.1a–c). He describes a colourful life, having been shipwrecked on an island for 26 years. He is accompanied by his friend, Friday, whom he consents to being present in the consultation. He is concerned as Friday has noticed a lesion on his scalp. He has recently seen a TV advert advising people who have had sun exposure and funny lesions to seek medical help. He said that on the island he was repeatedly sunburnt and had chronic sun exposure, and he has been bald for years. You notice a few lesions on his head, which are thickened yellow plaques. They are non tender.

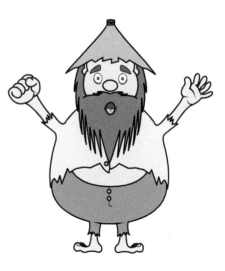

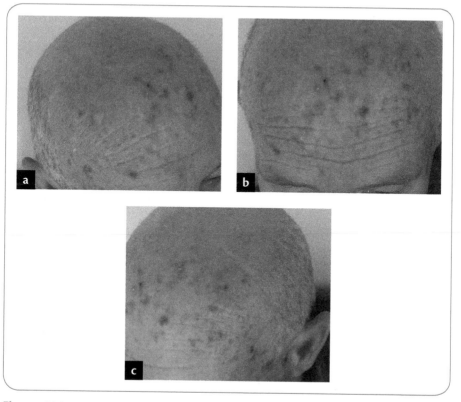

Figures 31.1a–c.

i. What do the pictures show?

They show actinic keratosis lesions, also known as solar keratosis. This is a precancerous form of squamous cell carcinoma, more common in the elderly. Risk factors for developing actinic keratosis include chronic sun exposure, fair skin and immunosuppression. It is important to ask about travel occupation, as patients who have had spent large amounts of time in the sun, such as gardeners or those who grew up in hot climates, are particularly at risk.

ii. What are the treatment options for actinic keratoses?

Treatment is largely for cosmetic reasons or if the lesions become uncomfortable. Because of the risk of them becoming malignant, they are often removed. Cryotherapy, curettage or local excision can be used to try and remove these lesions. Topical therapies are also used but this can cause local reactions, including inflammation and blistering, as illustrated in the pictures, which show these lesions post topical therapy where they become quite red. High factor sunscreen can help treat pre-existing lesions but the best preventive measures include good sun protection (avoid the midday sun, regular application of sunscreen, wear a hat, etc).

iii. What is the ABCDE rule of suspicious lesions?

This pneumonic is helpful when diagnosing melanomas, although a high index of suspicion should always be present and any uncertainty should be referred to a dermatologist:

A – asymmetry

B – border irregularity

C – colour, especially uneven colour within a lesion or a lesion different in colour to others

D – diameter >6 mm

E – evolving over time

OUTCOME

RC was treated with fluorourcil and had a local reaction for several weeks. He found life back in civilization hard to adjust to and was later arrested after the mysterious disappearance of his friend Friday, next to a large cooking pot.

CASE 32

Your consultant asks you to go and give your new Foundation doctor, Dr Reaper, a hand. He has been bleeped repeatedly by the bereavement office as there is a backlog of death certificates to complete following his weekend on call on the geriatric wards. On arrival to the bereavement office, you find Grim looking very stressed, surrounded by patient notes. You also make a mental note to discuss Grim's health with his supervisor, as he seems very skinny and withdrawn.

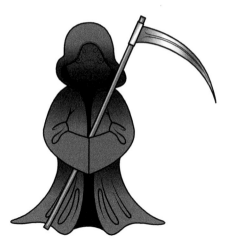

i. What should you document when confirming a death?

Confirming a patient has died forms part of the workload for junior doctors on the wards. Death is usually said to occur in an unresponsive patient who shows no signs of respiratory effort, has no cardiac output (measured by heart sounds and pulses), an absent corneal reflex and the pupils are fixed and dilated.

After checking with the nursing staff the circumstances around the death and confirming the identity, it is important to document your findings (Fig. 32.1):

Day, Date, & Time	
29/12/17	G. Reaper (F1)
03:40	Asked to confirm death.
	Patient is unresponsive.
	Patient has no breath sounds for 2 minutes
	Patient has no heart sounds or pulse for 2 minutes
	Patient has an absent corneal reflex and pupils are fixed and dilated
	No pacemaker noted
	Patient confirmed dead @ 03.40 on the 29th December 2017
	Rest in Peace A.N. Example
	G. Reaper
	F1 Medicine

Affix patient label
Hosp No. 0195
A.N. Example 23/3/1909

Figure 32.1.

ii. Why do we check for a pacemaker?

If a patient is to be cremated, it is important to check and document whether a pacemaker is palpated. This is because a part of some pacemakers can explode when exposed to extreme heat and this can damage the crematorium chambers. It is normally the mortician or funeral directors who would remove these.

iii. What cases need to be discussed with a coroner?

In some instances, the death of a patient needs to be discussed with the coroner. While each coroner will vary slightly and the list below is not exhaustive, commonly the following deaths that are reported include:

- Death within 24 hours of admission.
- Suicide or suspected suicide.
- Deaths of children and people under 18.
- Deaths that may be linked to medical treatment or recent operations (policies vary but often within 6 months).
- Deaths that may be linked to an accident.
- Deaths that are suspicious or violent in nature.
- Deaths related to industrial diseases (such as asbestos) or occupation.
- Death of any patient in custody or detained under the Mental Health Act (even if natural causes).

It is advised that you discuss the patient with a consultant prior to completing a death certificate and also discuss with the coroner, as they will be able to guide you. While this task can seem quite daunting, it is often merely a formality where you speak to the coroner's officer who will run the case past the coroner. If, for example, an 85 year old came in with sepsis and died within 24 hours but you had no cause for concern, you would need to report this to the coroner; however, it is likely they would say you could issue the death certificate without the need for a post mortem. Note that the coroner's decision is final and they can order a post mortem even if you do not think it is indicated.

OUTCOME

Dr Reaper completed the death certificates and one or two cremation forms, receiving the cremation form fee (also known as 'ash cash') a few weeks later. He loved watching Poldark on the television and so used his money to buy a scythe.

CASE 33

You are asked to see a patient in the emergency department who is making a lot of noise. The Hatter has come in with his friend, the March Hare, and a lost looking girl called Alice. The March Hare explains that they were just having a nice cup of tea when the Hatter started rambling and talking nonsensically about time. When speaking with the Hatter, he seems to jump from one idea to another and believes someone, the 'Queen of Hearts,' is out to kill him and wants to cut off his head. He speaks in riddles and keeps reciting poetry. The Hare is unsure about the Hatter's past medical history but thinks he may have a background of schizophrenia. The Hatter becomes increasingly agitated and starts becoming aggressive, breaking up items in the room and cutting himself on a smashed clock.

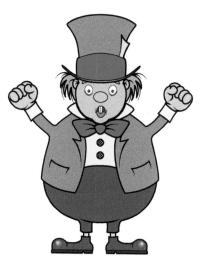

i. How do you assess capacity?

A patient is always assumed to have capacity. Note that a patient does not lack capacity if they simply make a 'bad decision' or one with which health professionals do not agree. It is necessary at times to assess a patient's capacity. A patient who lacks capacity must have an impairment of the functioning of their mind that affects their ability to make a decision. Under the Mental Health Act 1983, a person is regarded as being unable to make a decision if they cannot do the following (Fig. 33.1):

It is important that this is clearly documented in the notes, and policies between hospitals vary. Once a patient is deemed as lacking capacity, then health professionals can act in their best interests. Note that this is decision specific.

Criteria that a patient must fulfil to be regarded as unable to make a decision	
Unable to understand the information relevant to a decision	'Listen'
Unable to retain the information relevant to a decision	'Retain'
Unable to weigh the information	'Process'
Unable to communicate this decision	'Communicate'

Figure 33.1.

ii. Which sections of the Mental Health Act 1983 are commonly used by medical professionals and the police?

This is not only a favourite exam question, but is also important to know, as the legal implications are important (Fig. 33.2).

Section	Reason	Time	Who can perform this?
2	Assessment	Max 28 days	Started by a relative or mental health practitioner and two registered medical practitioners
3	Treatment	<6 months	
4	Emergency treatment	<72 hours	One registered medical practitioner
5 (2)	Patient an inpatient	<72 hours	One registered medical practitioner
5 (4)	Patient an inpatient	<6 hours	One registered nurse
135	Taken from private premises to place of safety	<72 hours	Police
136	Taken from public place to place of safety	<72 hours	Police

Figure 33.2.

iii. What is the difference between Gillick and Fraser competence?

The capacity assessment above relates to adults. When assessing if a child has the capacity to make a decision, the terms Gillick and Fraser are often referred to. Gillick competency stems from a case in 1982, where Mrs Gillick took her local health authority to court. The case arose due to a dispute as to whether an under 16 year old could make decisions regarding contraceptive advice and treatment. The outcome of the case was that if a child is mature enough and can understand the nature of the consent required, and if the child can make a reasonable assessment of the advantages and disadvantages of the treatment proposed, then it can be deemed true consent. This has led to the term, 'Gillick competent', which means the practitioner deems them mature enough to consent to the medical treatment or intervention. There is a myth that Mrs Gillick did not want her name used, hence the reason why Fraser is used interchangeably; however, they are different and should not be confused.

The Fraser guidelines refer to the guidelines made by Lord Fraser in his judgement of the case regarding contraceptive advice only. They outline that:

1. The girl will understand the advice.
2. They cannot be persuaded to inform their parents.
3. They will likely carry on sexual intercourse with or without the treatment.

4. Their physical or mental health will likely suffer unless they receive contraceptive advice or treatment.

5. It is in her best interests to give advice or treatment without the parental consent.

It is important to remember that children under the age of 13 cannot lawfully consent to sexual activity; this would be classified as rape, and so the Gillick test would not apply here.

OUTCOME

The Hatter was sectioned and after excluding a medical cause for his symptoms, he was transferred to the local psychiatric unit. He engaged well with the mental health team, enjoying their regular tea parties and was discharged back to the care of the March Hare eventually. He studied hard and became a Mental Health nurse himself.

CASE 34

Bob Cratchit, a local clerk, brings in his son Tim, an 11-month-old boy, to the GP one cold December morning. He has had a cough and a runny nose for about 2 days now, but over the past 12 hours his breathing has deteriorated. He was born prematurely at 36 weeks and you notice he was quite Tiny on his growth charts. He has only been managing just under half his normal fluid intake and has had about half of his normal wet nappies. There are several other children at home who have recently been unwell with a viral illness. You know

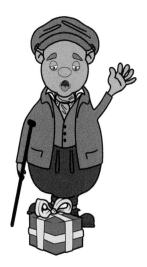

the family well and remember they are one of the Government's 'just about managing' families and Mr Cratchit is unkempt. On examination, Tim is afebrile, his heart rate is 160, RR is 40 and he has moderate intercostal recession. There are widespread crackles on auscultation. You suspect that Tim has bronchiolitis.

i. What is bronchiolitis?

Bronchiolitis is an inflammation of the bronchioles in a young baby or infant. It is an acute infectious disease, usually occurring in children younger than 2 but that has a peak in babies between 3 and 6 months, and it has seasonal variation. On a paediatric ward, staff may mention 'bronc season' as the ward can have lots of patients suffering with this. It is mainly a viral illness and is most often caused by the respiratory syncytial virus (RSV) but others, including adenovirus, parainfluenza virus and coronavirus, may also cause the disease. Younger children and those born prematurely or small for age and with other co-morbidities are more at risk, and parental smoking and those with an older sibling that attends nursery also increases the risk. Approximately 1 in 3 children will develop clinical bronchiolitis in the first year of life; however, for most of these, it is a self-limiting illness with only about 2% of these requiring hospitalization. It normally presents with increased work of breathing, coryzal symptoms, poor feeding and often widespread crackles on auscultation. Apnoea may be the presenting feature in younger children. A fever above 39°C is unusual and should point towards an alternative diagnosis. Days 3–5 can be the peak of the illness and the cough can last about 2 weeks.

ii. What are the normal observation values for children?

Although this is difficult to retain, it is worth being aware of the different values of vital signs for children and having these as a quick reference in your GP practice or emergency department. They vary depending on the resource; a guide is shown below (Fig. 34.1).

Age (years)	Heart rate	Respiratory rate	Systolic blood pressure
<1	110–160	30–40	70–90
1–2	100–150	25–35	80–95
2–5	95–140	25–30	80–100
5–12	80–120	20–25	90–110
Over 12	60–100	15–20	100–120

Figure 34.1.

Parental concern or healthcare professional concern should also be taken into account as a marker of how unwell a patient is, and this should not be underestimated.

iii. What would warrant a review by the paediatric team?

There are many traffic light systems used to try and stratify risk for patients. One is shown below (**Fig. 34.2**). The main criteria for admission are the need for

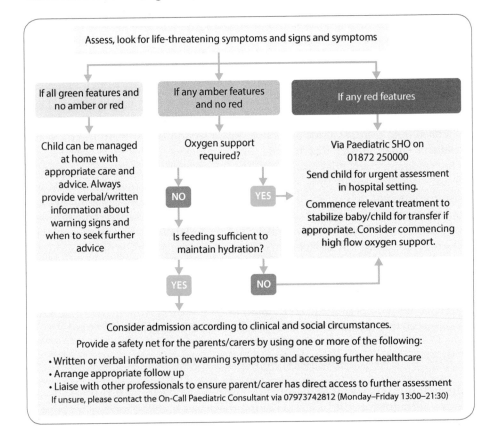

Figure 34.2.

oxygen support (determined largely by oxygen saturations) and for feeding support (whether fluid challenges or nasogastric [NG] feeding). Feeding is important to take into consideration as due to the fast respiratory rate, patients can find it difficult to get enough oral intake. This can be likened to trying to drink while running and out of breath. A patient having less than 50% of their feed would need review and likely need NG feeding.

OUTCOME

Tiny Tim was admitted to the ward where he received supplementary oxygen and NG feeding. A nasopharyngeal aspirate confirmed RSV. He improved slowly. Mr Cratchit was very distressed by his need for admission as he felt his boss, Mr Scrooge, would fire him if he did not turn up to work and he had been trying to save money to buy a Christmas present for each of his children. However, Scrooge turned up to the ward on Christmas Eve just prior to discharge dressed as Father Christmas and bought all of Mr Cratchit's children presents and a large Christmas turkey.

CASE 35

A 17-year-old girl doing some work experience on the ward as part of her royal duties presents to the accident and emergency department with a needle-stick injury. You are struck by how beautiful she is. She is quite shy and keeps yawning. One of the staff accompanying her tells you that she pricked herself on an old spindle on the ward. On examination she has a small puncture wound on the end of her finger.

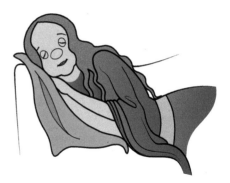

i. What is a needlestick injury?

A needlestick injury is an injury caused by penetration from a sharp instrument or needle. If this needle is contaminated with infected blood, then there is a potential for this to be transmitted to the injured person. Although there is a risk of passing any infectious organism, the main concerns are HIV, hepatitis B and hepatitis C.

ii. What should you do as a medical professional if you sustain a needlestick injury?

Needlestick injuries are unfortunately common in the NHS and form one of the largest causes of injury (behind manual handling). You should always be open and honest about an injury and it is important to remember you will not get into trouble for getting one – accidents do happen! Most Trusts have a 'needlestick bleep' where advice can be gained 24 hours a day. If you sustain a needlestick injury you should wash your hand under a running tap for several minutes. Each hospital varies but on wards there may be an Inoculation Injury Kit (Fig. 35.1) with the equipment and

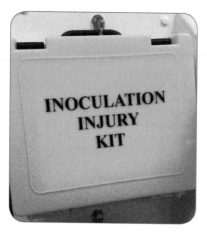

Figure 35.1.

guidance needed to manage the injury. It is important to keep a note of the patient details whose blood you have been contaminated with, as their risk of blood-borne viruses will need to be assessed and, with their consent, a sample taken and tested.

iii. How can you prevent needlestick injuries in the workplace?

Needlestick injuries are more common in staff that are tired, overstretched or distracted, therefore ensure when performing a procedure that all steps are taken to reduce the risk of injury, including handing a bleep to a colleague. Sharps should be disposed of in a designated sharps bin (Fig. 35.2). It is important not to fill the bins up above the line. Sharps should not be carried around the ward. Needles should not be re-sheathed after use.

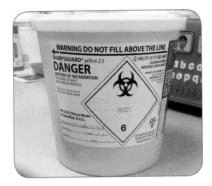

Figure 35.2.

Needles with guards on them (Fig. 35.3) have been introduced on many wards; however, they have not been shown to drastically reduce incidents and indeed may cause more injury due to splashes when trying to close the guard.

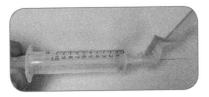

Figure 35.3.

OUTCOME

The patient is referred to occupational health. En route, she collapses into a deep sleep and this coma lasts nearly a hundred years. A handsome prince visits her one day on the ward during the opening of a new wing in the hospital. He kisses her as he feels that she is so beautiful and she starts to open her eyes and is extubated. When she finally comes out of her coma, she returns to the department to give you a thank you card. She finds that you are still working as they have moved the retirement age further and further.

CASE 36

A young girl in a red cloak is brought into the emergency department. She was walking alone in the woods when she was attacked by a big bad wolf and has bite wounds to her forearm. Her mother has brought her in as she thinks she needs stitches.

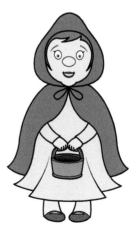

i. Should you close the wounds?

No. Animal and human bites are contaminated wounds due to the organisms carried in the mouth and they have a high rate of infection if they are sutured directly. Appropriate management is cleaning the wound, examining for any evidence of damage to the underlying structures (nerves/blood vessels/tendons), ensuring tetanus status is up to date, antibiotic prophylaxis and referring the patient for appropriate debridement of the wounds in the operating theatre.

ii. What organisms are commonly responsible for infections after animal bites?

Dog bites commonly contain multiple aerobic and anaerobic organisms, with *Pasturella* species being the most common. Cat bites have a similar spectrum of microorganisms to dogs; however, in human bites streptococci and *Eikenella corrodens* are more common.

iii. What underlying structures are at risk?

Any structures within the zone of injury are at risk and these should all be examined clinically before any treatment is carried out. In the forearm it is vital to examine the motor and sensory functions of the median, ulna and radial nerves, look for any evidence of damage to the radial or ulnar arteries and examine individually the isolated function of each underlying muscle or tendon.

OUTCOME

The girl returned home after having her wounds explored and cleaned in the operating theatre and they healed uneventfully. The wolf was reported to the local authorities and was detained under the Dangerous Dogs Act 1991. It was later destroyed and everyone else lived happily ever after.

CASE 37

A small child is carried into your department. He has been using a crutch for some time and is complaining of right-sided hip pain but has been unable to visit you as his father has been so busy at work.

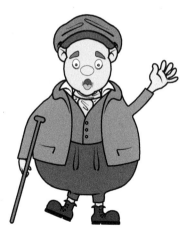

i. What are the differential diagnoses of hip pain in a child?

There are many potential causes of atraumatic hip pain. Septic arthritis can occur in any age and is often seen in accompaniment with fever, an inability to weight bear, raised inflammatory markers and an unwell child. Transient synovitis can mimic infection, but is an inflammatory disorder most often triggered by a recent viral illness. In the older child a slipped upper femoral epiphysis can be the cause, starting around puberty and usually necessitating surgical pinning. Perthes disease of the hip can occur usually between the ages of 4 and 8 years.

ii. What is Perthes disease of the hip?

Perthes disease is idiopathic avascular necrosis of the hip. There is no known cause or trigger but the condition generally begins between the ages of 4 and 8 and, as with any disorder of the hip joint, can present with referred pain in the knee. Radiographs show flattening and later fragmentation of the femoral head and treatment is aimed at protecting the weight-bearing across the hip, although surgery is sometimes required.

iii. What other bones are vulnerable to avascular necrosis?

Avascular necrosis is ischaemia and death of bone due to an interruption in its blood supply. Causes include trauma, steroids and alcohol. Sites classically affected include the femoral head, scaphoid and the talus, as their blood supply is especially vulnerable.

OUTCOME

The child was diagnosed with Perthes disease and treated with physiotherapy, with good outcome due to his young age. He went on to have many happy Christmases.

CASE 38

An American millionaire engineer visits you complaining of lethargy. He has been increasingly tired and finding it difficult to work as a crime fighting superhero. He tells you his father suffered from a similar problem. You remove his heavy metal suit to examine him and note a slate grey colour of the skin. After a thorough systemic examination, you suspect a diagnosis of haemochromatosis.

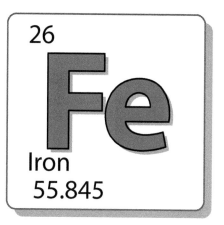

26

Fe

Iron

55.845

i. What is haemochromatosis?

This is a condition of iron overload, which may be genetically acquired in an autosomal recessive manner or result from iron accumulation from repeated blood transfusions. It is particularly common in northern European ancestry, especially Celtic descent. As iron accumulates in the body, it is deposited in the tissues as haemosiderin, which is toxic by inducing oxidative stress. Haemochromatosis is diagnosed by serum ferritin and transferrin saturation levels.

ii. What are the systemic complications?

Common organs affected include: the liver, causing cirrhosis; bones and joints, causing arthritis; skin, causing a grey or bronze pigmentation; pancreas, causing diabetes mellitus; heart, causing cardiac failure, arrhythmias or pericarditis; and adrenal glands, causing adrenal insufficiency.

iii. How can the condition be managed?

Management is aimed at preventing the accumulation of iron and therefore organ damage in the early stages of disease. This is most easily achieved by periodic venesection at regular intervals. When this is not possible, desferrioxamine mesilate can be used as an iron chelating agent to induce excretion of iron. In later stages, end organ damage may also require management such as ACE inhibitors for heart failure and insulin for diabetes.

OUTCOME

The gentleman was diagnosed with haemochromatosis and placed on a regular monitoring and blood letting regime. Unfortunately, he was lost to follow up as he was too busy fighting multinational crime to attend regular clinic appointments. He subsequently developed liver cirrhosis and was no longer able to get into his crime fighting suit due to stiff painful joints and tense ascites.

CASE 39

A beautiful princess presents to the Royal Hospital, accompanied by seven of her friends, all short in stature and carrying a variety of garden implements. Her friends report that the patient has ingested an unknown substance, given to her by an old woman, together with some alcohol. The police are involved as they have so far been unable to corroborate this story and had suspected the use of Rohypnol (flunitrazepam). She had apparently been quite low in mood recently after some bad dates she had been on with 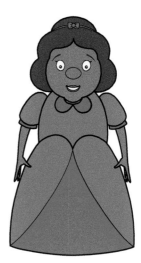 unsuitable suitors. The police found a diary stating that she might end her life if she were not to find love. After ingesting this substance she later had a seizure lasting a few minutes. This involved her arms and legs shaking violently and foaming at the mouth. There is no evidence of incontinence or tongue biting and one of the friends said she was blue around her lips and fingers. Since then she has seemed to be fast asleep.

The police searched the property and stated that there was no other paraphernalia found, apart from a half eaten apple core. She has no known medical conditions and no allergies that they are aware of. She is normally fit and well.

On initial presentation to the hospital wing, her oxygen saturations were 99% on room air with equal entry on both sides and no chest crackles. She was snoring quite loudly but a simple head tilt chin lift resolved this and a nasopharyngeal airway was inserted easily. There was no clinical evidence of aspiration. Her heart rate was regular, pulse rate 135, BP 110/65 with normal heart sounds. Her GCS was E2, V3, M5 = 10/15. Her pupils were dilated but reactive.

A bedside glucose was 8.5 mmol/L; a portable chest radiograph did not reveal any signs of aspiration. A blood gas showed a pH of 7.28, PaCO$_2$ of 34 mmHg and an HCO$_3$ of 19 mEq/L. A toxicology screen was negative and her paracetamol levels were in the normal range. An ECG demonstrated a sinus tachycardia with prolonged QT interval and a widened QRS complex.

i. What does the blood gas show?

The blood gas shows a metabolic acidosis, with some compensation. Interpretation of the blood gases is shown in the Table (Fig. 39.1).

ABG result	pH (normal 7.35–7.45)	PaCO₂ (normal 35–45 mmHg)	HCO₃ (22–28 mEq/L)
Respiratory acidosis	↓	↑	Normal
Respiratory alkalosis	↑	↓	Normal
Metabolic acidosis	↓	Normal	↓
Metabolic alkalosis	↑	Normal	↑
Respiratory acidosis with some metabolic compensation	↓	↑	↑
Metabolic acidosis with some respiratory compensation	↓	↓	↓

Figure 39.1.

ii. What drug would you be worried about that prolongs QT intervals and causes a widened QRS complex?

In this case, there is a high suspicion of a tricyclic antidepressant overdose due to the ECG changes and the seizure activity. This can cause antimuscarinic effects such as tachycardia, blurred vision, dry mouth and urinary retention. Patients may go on to develop hypotension and arrhythmias and so cardiac monitoring is essential. Life-threatening events tend to occur within the first 6 hours of ingestion.

iii. What is the treatment of this case?

As with all situations in the emergency department, a systematic approach, using the ABCDE approach, will ensure that a thorough prioritized assessment is made. Sodium bicarbonate may be given to correct the metabolic acidosis together with hyperventilation if ventilation is required. Indications for sodium bicarbonate in tricyclic overdose include a widened QRS, seizures or hypotension not responsive to fluids.

OUTCOME

The patient improved quickly on the unit and was transferred to the female ward of the castle. It was never discovered exactly what she had taken but she was referred to the Mental Health Services and was discharged, with liaison with the drugs and alcohol team. She then later went on to make a full recovery and married her charming prince. All charges were dropped against her friends.

CASE 40

A mermaid presents to your GP clinic. She had refused to see the male medical student. She is a bit embarrassed and after some excellent use of Pendleton's consultation model, you elicit that she is suffering from a vaginal discharge. She describes this as smelling strongly of fish. She becomes a bit tearful as she says that she recently had sexual intercourse with a handsome prince and is worried that he has been unfaithful to her. You send a sample to the lab who say there is a positive 'whiff' test and the presence of clue cells.

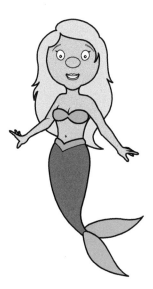

i. What is your differential diagnosis?

The common causes of vaginitis and discharge are listed in the Fig. 40.1.

Given the offensive 'fishy' discharge, you should suspect a diagnosis of bacterial vaginosis (BV). Both BV and trichomoniasis can present quite similarly and so it can be difficult to separate the two diagnoses. A positive 'whiff' test is performed by adding potassium hydroxide to the sample, which results in a strong fishy/alkaline smell. This can be positive in both BV and trichomoniasis. However, under a microscope, the presence of 'clue' cells points towards a diagnosis of BV. 'Clue' cells are vaginal epithelial cells covered in gram-negative rods, pathognomonic for BV.

	Discharge	Other symptoms
Candida (thrush)	'Cottage cheese'	Vulvitis, itch
Bacterial vaginosis	Offensive, thin, milky white, 'fishy odour'	Odour can be worse after intercourse
Trichomonas vaginalis	Offensive, green, frothy discharge	Itching, strawberry cervix
Chlamydia	May have no discharge	Dysuria, bleeding after sex. Often asymptomatic

Figure 40.1.

ii. What are the Amsel criteria?

The Amsel criteria are shown below. The presence of any three of the criteria would point towards a diagnosis of BV:

1. Vaginal pH greater than 4.5.
2. Positive 'whiff' test (see above).
3. Presence of clue cells.
4. Thin, homogeneous discharge.

iii. What is the treatment of this condition?

Treatment of BV is with antibiotics. Local protocols may vary but usually metronidazole is used first line.

OUTCOME

The Little Mermaid completed a course of metronidazole. She was pleased to know that BV was not likely sexually transmitted and continued to be besotted with the prince. She found it hard to adapt to life on the mainland and was referred to gynaecology as she couldn't seem to get rid of her fishy odour and several infestations of crabs.

CASE 41

Bambi comes into your GP office one morning complaining of a rash, lethargy and feeling like he has the flu. He recently lost his mother during a violent attack when she was shot and he has been to see you a few times with symptoms of low mood, for which he takes citalopram and is receiving cognitive behavioural therapy. He has no allergies and is otherwise fit and well. He reports having been on a stag do about a week ago in the New Forest. On the stag do, they went paintballing and

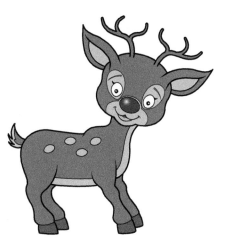

he noticed he had a tick bite, which he removed. Despite removing this, he says the rash has spread. He does not have a fever currently and his observations are all within normal range. On examination he has a rash on his left thigh approximately 5.5 cm in diameter. There is an area of erythema at the site of the tick bite, surrounded by a paler area with a ring of erythema surrounding this that he says is spreading.

i. What is the likely diagnosis?

Given the history of a tick bite and this characteristic rash, the most likely cause of this patient's symptoms is Lyme disease. Lyme disease is an infectious disease that is caused by *Borrelia burgdorferi* (a spirochaete). It is common in Europe and North America. It is spread by ticks. It is more common in areas of larger deer populations and is thought to be increasing in incidence in the UK, especially in the South of England and the Scottish Highlands. Apart from the rash, which approximately 20% of patients may not have, symptoms include a flu-like illness. Later some people may develop a facial palsy, meningitis, arthritis or carditis. (Matt Dawson, the former England rugby player, needed cardiac surgery following a tick bite.). There is increasing evidence of a post-infectious Lyme disease that has a lot of overlap with signs of fibromyalgia.

ii. What is the name of this rash?

The rash described sounds like erythema migrans. This is a red and expanding rash that can follow a tick bite. It can appear on average 7–10 days post bite and, as explained above, not all patients with Lyme disease will have this rash. The rash starts at the site of the tick bite as an erythematous macule. This is surrounded by a clearer area that is itself surrounded by a spreading erythematous ring. This gives it its characteristic 'bullseye' appearance (Fig. 41.1).

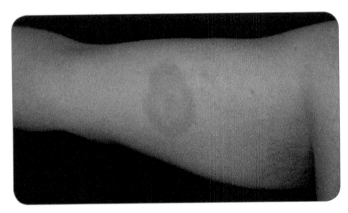

Figure 41.1.

iii. What is the treatment for Lyme disease?

The treatment of Lyme disease varies between areas but often doxycycline, amoxicillin or cefuroxime are used first line and are often needed for 2 weeks. Course length may be longer and intravenous treatment may be needed for complications including facial palsy.

OUTCOME

Bambi completed a 3-week course of doxycycline and reported that his symptoms were much improved. He continued to be troubled with low mood following the death of his mother and unfortunately was involved in a motor vehicle accident at night, when he was crossing the road.

CASE 42

You get a pre-alert call regarding a 32-year-old male frog who was involved in a road traffic collision while driving when intoxicated in his vintage car near his manor house. They tell you he is comatose, has low BP and a deformed right arm and leg.

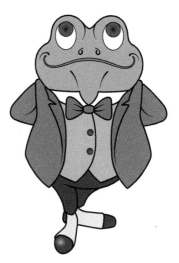

i. How is major trauma managed initially?

Major trauma in the UK is usually diverted directly to a major trauma unit for initial assessment and management. Here patients are greeted by a multidisciplinary trauma team and assessed and treated. The Advanced Trauma Life Support system is used to assess patients and identify major threats to life. It involves assessing and managing airway problems along with immobilising the cervical spine first, assessing and managing breathing problems next followed by circulatory problems then disability and exposure. In reality these sequences are all performed in tandem by different members of the trauma team.

ii. What is permissive hypotension?

This is the concept that in hypotensive patients clots are formed in bleeding vessels that prevent further blood loss. With overly aggressive resuscitation to restore normal BP, these clots may be disrupted, leading to further blood loss. Instead patients should be resuscitated to a low-normal BP using warmed blood and blood products instead of crystalloid. These are available through activating the local major haemorrhage protocol.

iii. When should surgery be performed for long bone fractures?

Major trauma causes activation of the systemic inflammatory response syndrome. A further surgical insult can exacerbate this further and lead to worse outcomes. Damage control surgery is a concept that in critically unwell patients, fast temporary surgery is used to stabilize fractures while minimizing this second insult. This is usually through the use of external fixators with definitive surgery undertaken once the systemic inflammatory response has settled.

This decision is made on a variety of factors including vital signs, blood gas readings and plasma lactate concentration. In patients who are physiologically stable, early total care may be used to definitively fix each injury early in order to allow single surgery and earlier mobilization.

OUTCOME

After arrival in the emergency department the patient was intubated, put in a pelvic binder, resuscitated with blood products and sent to theatre for stabilization of the limb fractures with external fixators. He made a prolonged but good recovery, although he still has a croaky voice. He continues his love for fast cars, lily ponds and high-class prostitutes.

CASE 43

An alien from outer space is brought to the emergency department by a child. He has a red hot glowing fingertip on the index finger of his left hand. You try to examine the finger, but the alien insists on making a phone call first. The patient is afebrile but has a tender red swelling over the fingertip. You suspect an infective process.

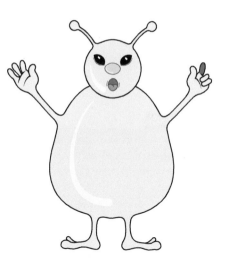

i. What are the different types of infection possible in the finger?

Cellulitis of the hand is a superficial soft tissue infection often caused by staphylococcal or streptococcal species. If there is collection of pus adjacent to the nail, this is called a paronychia. An infection or collection of pus in the fingertip pulp is called a felon and is usually caused by a penetrating injury. Penetrating injuries around the flexor tendons of the fingers can also cause infection of the flexor sheath. As in all infective processes, where there is a collection of pus, this must be drained for resolution of infection to occur.

ii. How do you identify a flexor sheath infection?

A penetrating injury to the volar aspect of the finger should raise suspicion for this condition. Classically, this is caused by a thorn while gardening. While examining the patient there are four cardinal signs, described by Kanavel and all suggestive of a flexor sheath infection, to look out for:

1. Fusiform swelling of the whole digit.
2. A flexed posture of the finger.
3. Pain on passive extension of the digit.
4. Palmar tenderness over the flexor sheath.

iii. Why is flexor sheath infection important to diagnose?

Flexion of the fingers is vital for everyday function. When infection occurs untreated in a tight space such as the flexor sheath this can lead to necrosis and scarring. Scarring of the flexor tendons will lead to significant functional impairment such as an inability to make a fist or grasp objects. In addition, the sheathes of the little and index finger are often continuous at the wrist and infection to one can spread to the other in a so called 'horseshoe abscess'. It is important that infections of the flexor sheath are treated early with surgical irrigation of the flexor sheath as well as intravenous antibiotics and elevation of the limb.

OUTCOME

You suspected a paronychia and performed an incision and drainage under digital block in the emergency department. You later received a call from the microbiologist to inform you that samples had grown a super-infectious alien microorganism. The whole hospital had to be evacuated for quarantine and an extensive 'deep-clean', while the patient was repatriated to his home planet where the appropriate antibiotics exist to ensure a successful recovery.

CASE 44

A gentleman attends the emergency department along with his friends, a young girl and a cowardly lion. He tells you he had been having significant pain and a creaking sensation on walking. This had been especially bad recently as he has been on a long journey along a yellow paved road. He has previously had multiple operations including bilateral hip, knee, ankle, shoulder and elbow replacements, which were done for osteoarthritis. He

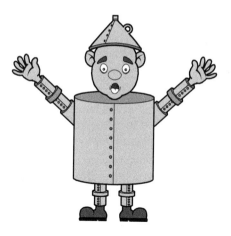

tells you these were done with tin implants. He has come for a routine check-up following the most recent left hip replacement. You find him well; his wound has healed and he is walking comfortably without aid.

i. What are the radiological signs of osteoarthritis?

These can be remembered using the mnemonic 'LOSS', which represent **L**oss of joint space, **O**steophytes, **S**ubchondral sclerosis and **S**ubchondral cysts (Fig. 44.1). The signs of inflammatory arthritis, such as rheumatoid arthritis, differ. Here soft tissue swelling, periarticular osteopenia and periarticular erosions predominate as well as narrowing of the joint space (Fig. 44.2).

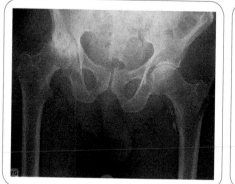

Figure 44.1.

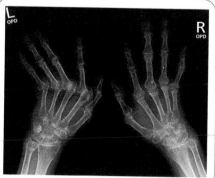

Figure 44.2.

ii. What are the treatment options in general for osteoarthritis?

Simple treatment begins with analgesia and lifestyle modification. This consists of simple painkillers like paracetamol and anti-inflammatories such as ibuprofen. Weight loss helps reduce joint reaction forces on weight-bearing joints and will aid symptoms. Bracing or splinting may help depending on the joint involved, and even intra-articular injection of steroid and local anaesthetic can be given to give temporary relief of an acute flare-up. When these methods fail there are three major categories of surgical options, dependent on the joint involved and patient factors:

1. Osteotomy involves cutting the bone and realigning the mechanical axis of the joint to offload contact pressures on the degenerative portion of the joint; it is usually used in early disease and young patients.

2. Arthrodesis (fusion) involves removing the joint surface and making the bones around the joint heal to each other to relieve pain at the expense of movement. This is commonly used in the hand and ankle.

3. Arthroplasty is removal of the joint with interposition of another material in the joint space such as a hip or knee prosthesis. This is common in the hip and knee and has excellent results in relieving pain whilst preserving movement.

iii. Are there any complications of joint replacements?

Of course, all surgical procedures come with potential complications. Infection of any prosthetic material is possible and is difficult to eradicate due to biofilm formation. Blood loss during large joint replacements may require blood transfusion. There are structures at risk in each joint replacement, such as the sciatic nerve in the hip or the popliteal structures in the knee. Venous thromboembolism is a risk, especially in surgery of the pelvis or lower limb, and necessitates thromboprophylaxis in the postoperative period. All prostheses are subject to wear and loosening over time, which may necessitate major revision surgery. In addition, there may be a risk of dislocation, especially in the hip, and change in leg length.

OUTCOME

The patient was very happy with the outcome of the procedure and was keen to get more mobile to go on a journey in search for a heart. You administered an intra-articular injection of WD40 to his remaining joints and he felt much less creaky and was very happy. Despite this you place him on the metal-on-metal surveillance programme where he receives regular check ups of his implants.

CASE 45

The Caterpillar comes into your GP clinic accompanied by his friend the Hatter. He is a lifelong smoker and you suspect he also partakes in magic mushrooms. He reports that he smokes nearly constantly throughout the day with a pipe. He reports coughing up phlegm everyday; however, in the past 2 days he reports the phlegm has changed colour to a dark brown/yellow. He is also coughing up much more than normal and feels fever-

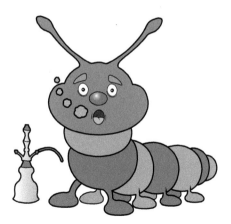

ish and unwell. You note he has a previous diagnosis of chronic obstructive pulmonary disease (COPD) and depression. He has no allergies. He currently takes a salbutamol inhaler. On examination, his oxygen saturations are 87% in air, respiratory rate is 35, temperature 38.1°C, there are signs of clubbing on his hands and on examination of his chest he has widespread wheeze.

i. What features would suggest an exacerbation of COPD?

It is often difficult to distinguish between a non-infective and an infective exacerbation of COPD. Patients with COPD may have a productive cough normally, but an exacerbation would be suggested by an increase in the amount of sputum, a colour change, worsening breathlessness and cough or a deterioration in their normal state. A course of steroids is usually given to treat this, together with antibiotics if indicated. It is recommended that antibiotics be given in those patients with purulent sputum or signs of pneumonia. The most common organisms that cause bacterial exacer-bations of COPD are *Haemophilus influenzae*, *Streptococcus pneumoniae* and *Moraxella cattarhalis*. Nebulizers may be needed if the patient is very wheezy and struggling with breathlessness. It should be remembered that COPD still carries a significant mortality and patients requiring hospitalization may need non-invasive ventilation if they develop a significant respiratory acidosis and show signs of fatigue.

ii. What is the biggest factor in the history above that would improve the patient's long-term survival?

In patients with stable COPD, the single biggest intervention that can be done to improve survival is smoking cessation. This should be done with the help of primary care services and may include nicotine replacement therapy. It should also be remembered that there is a risk of fire with patients who smoke and have home oxygen, although interestingly this is not an absolute contraindication.

iii. What vaccinations should a patient with COPD receive?

Patients with COPD should be advised to have the annual influenza vaccine and also have a one-off pneumococcal vaccination.

OUTCOME

The Caterpillar continued to smoke despite your advice and over the next few months had several exacerbations requiring hospital admissions. He was arrested by the Queen's men along with his friend the Hatter due to drug smuggling attempts and he was later sentenced to the guillotine.

CASE 46

Old Macdonald, a local farmer of pigs, cows, sheep, chickens and horses, presents to your GP practice. He was recently seen in the respiratory clinic for follow up for his pulmonary fibrosis. He recounts that years ago he was given a diagnosis of extrinsic allergic alveolitis and the nurse said this was caused by 'farmer's lung.' He has been reading on the internet that this is due to inhaling mouldy hay. He was told in the recent clinic follow up that his spirometry showed a restrictive pattern and he wants to know what this means. On examination, his saturations are 95% in room air, he has clubbing of his fingers and fine inspiratory crackles can be heard throughout the chest.

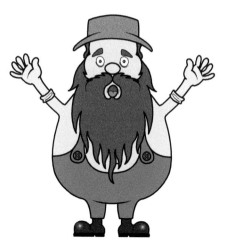

i. What is the difference between a restrictive and an obstructive spirometry test result?

Spirometry is a relatively cheap, non-invasive, readily available test used to assess lung function by measuring timed inspired and expired lung volumes. Spirometry results include FVC (forced vital capacity) and FEV1 (forced expiratory lung volume in 1 second). FVC is the total amount of air forcefully exhaled after the biggest breath possible, whilst FEV1 is the amount of air a person can forcefully exhale in one second (Fig. 46.1).

	Spirometry results	
	Obstructive lung disease	Restrictive lung disease
FEV1	Reduced	Reduced
FVC	Reduced or normal	Reduced
FEV1-FVC ratio	Reduced	Normal or increased

Figure 46.1.

ii. What are some of the common causes of both obstructive and restrictive lung diseases?

The causes of an obstructive pattern include: asthma, COPD, bronchiectasis and cystic fibrosis. The conditions causing restrictive lung disease include: pulmonary fibrosis, sarcoidosis, obesity, kyphoscoliosis, asbestosis and neuromuscular disease.

iii. What are the causes of clubbing?

There are numerous causes of this clinical sign and it is important to look for this as part of your clinical examination (Fig. 46.2).

	Causes of clubbing		
Cardiac causes	Bacterial endocarditis		
	Congenital cardiac disease		
	Atrial myxoma		
Respiratory causes	Lung cancer		
	Fibrosing alveolitis		
	Asbestosis		
	Tuberculosis		
	Cystic fibrosis		
	Sarcoidosis		
	Empyema		
	Interstitial lung disease		
	Idiopathic pulmonary fibrosis		
	Bronchiectais		
Other causes	Familial		
	Crohn's		
	Primary biliary corrhosis		
	Grave's disease		
	Pregnancy		

Figure 46.2.

OUTCOME

Mr McDonald was satisfied with the consultation and explanation provided to him. He continued to farm until he was very old indeed, but due to cuts in subsidies he diversified and converted some of his barns into holiday cottages. Despite being a staunch supporter of Britain leaving the EU, he frequently returned to your practice with signs of depression as he was worried about the future of the subsidies for local farmers. He also released a UK Number 1 Hit single about his animals, containing a chorus made up largely of vowels.

CASE 47

A mad professor approaches you while you are on your coffee break. He is very excited and through his garbled speech you decipher that he is telling you about a new screening test he has devised for serum rhubarb. He wants you to help him design a trial to prove evidence that his test will save countless lives through detecting this deadly vegetable toxin.

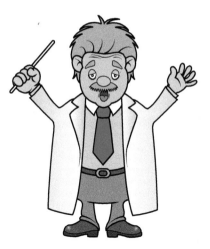

i. What are the different levels of evidence available?

When considering evidence based medicine it is important to stratify the different types of study according to the strength of the type of evidence and to what degree you can rely on that evidence to make decisions to change your practice or to base your treatment upon. The gold standard is a well-designed randomized control trial or systematic reviews of such trials. The lowest standard is expert opinion. All five levels are illustrated in the pyramid shown (**Fig. 47.1**).

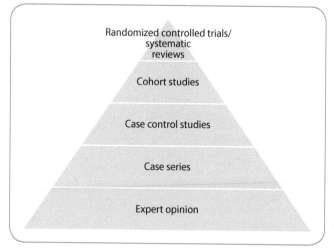

Randomized controlled trials/
systematic
reviews

Cohort studies

Case control studies

Case series

Expert opinion

Figure 47.1.

ii. How do you measure how well a test works?

Basic statistics are not only important when it comes to examinations but also to understanding research papers. The sensitivity of a test is a measure of how well a test can correctly identify those with the disease. The specificity of a test is a measure of how well the test can correctly identify those without the disease (Fig. 47.2).

	Has disease	Doesn't have disease
Test positive	True positive (TP)	False positive (FP)
Test negative	False negative (FN)	True negative (TN)

Figure 47.2.

Sensitivity (%) = (TP/TP + FN) × 100; specificity (%) = (TN/TN + FP) × 100.

iii. How do you decide if a disease is suitable for a screening programme?

The World Health Organization published the following guidelines on the principles of screening; these are commonly known as Wilson's criteria:

1. The condition should be an important health problem.
2. There should be a treatment for the condition.
3. Facilities for diagnosis and treatment should be available.
4. There should be a latent stage of the disease.
5. There should be a test or examination for the condition.
6. The test should be acceptable to the population.
7. The natural history of the disease should be adequately understood.
8. There should be an agreed policy on whom to treat.
9. The total cost of finding a case should be economically balanced in relation to medical expenditure as a whole.
10. Case-finding should be a continuous process, not just a 'once and for all' project.

OUTCOME

You help the author by setting up a rigorous trial with ethical approval to investigate the potential of this new test. After passing through all relevant trials the test is widely adopted worldwide and saves countless lives from dying of rhubarb toxaemia. The professor is nominated for the Nobel prize; however, despite your significant contribution to the work, he neglected to include your name as an author on the seminal paper. Your friends and colleagues are adamant that your frequent claims of your involvement are nothing but fantasy tales.

CASE 48

A young lady who goes by the name of Cindy is brought to the emergency department by her new boyfriend. She tells you she was trying on a new pair of glass slippers when she twisted awkwardly on her left ankle. The ankle has become swollen and bruised and she is unable to walk on that foot. You examine her and find some bruising and swelling on the lateral side of the ankle and you suspect an ankle sprain. Her boyfriend is very pushy and is insistent on her being radiographed.

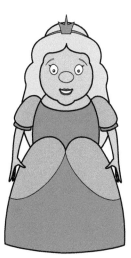

i. How do you decide who requires a radiograph of the ankle?

The Ottowa Ankle Rules are validated rules that state an ankle radiograph is required if the patient is unable to bear weight immediately and is in the emergency department or has bony tenderness over the posterior edge or tip of the medial or lateral malleolus in the distal 6 cm (Figs. 48.1a, b). Tenderness over the 5th metatarsal or navicular means a foot series should be performed.

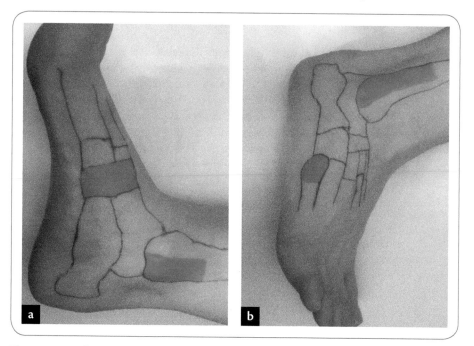

Figures 48.1a, b.

ii. What can you see in the radiograph (Fig. 48.2)?

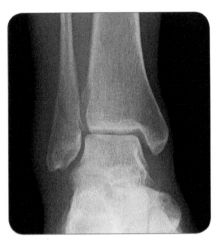

Figure 48.2.

The radiograph shows a spiral fracture of the fibula at the level of the ankle joint. This would be classified as a Weber B injury as the fracture is at the level of the syndesmosis. In Weber A injuries the fracture line is below the syndesmosis and in Weber C injuries the fracture line is above the syndesmosis. This helps predict injury to the syndesmosis and ankle stability.

iii. What are the treatment options for ankle fractures such as this?

Conservative treatment is suitable for non-displaced fractures that are stable. Protection can be provided in a below knee plaster or a walking boot and the patient should be followed up in the fracture clinic. For stable injuries patients should be allowed to bear weight as tolerated. Some people advocate thromboprophylaxis when immobilizing ankle fractures; however, there is no concrete evidence either way on the benefit of this. Unstable injuries where there is any disruption of the ankle joint, syndesmosis or a bimalleolar fracture are usually treated with internal fixation by an orthopaedic surgeon.

OUTCOME

You place Cindy in a below knee plaster and she leaves with her partner in a large pumpkin carriage. Unfortunately, she is unable to go to the upcoming ball due to her injury and her partner decides to take her stepsister instead. Although Cindy's fracture heals over the next few months, she suspects her boyfriend is having an affair with her more mobile stepsister. At her 6-month follow up appointment she is back working as a housemaid. She tells you her ex-boyfriend and stepsister have since married and she is seeking damages from her wealthy ex through a no win no fee legal team.

CASE 49

Achilles, a 25-year-old Greek gentleman, presents with pain in his heel and difficulty walking. He describes dodging a horse and cart while crossing a road after having attending the local steam baths. He felt a sudden pain to the back of the heel as if he was hit by someone. He did look around but there was no one in sight. He is unable to stand on his tip toes and you feel a palpable gap at the back of his heel. You suspect an Achilles tendon rupture.

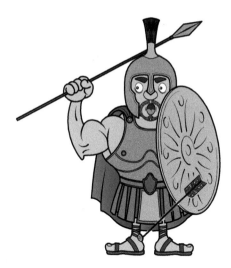

i. What bedside test can be used to aid diagnosis?

An Achilles tendon rupture is a clinical diagnosis based on the history and examination, especially the calf squeeze test. This is also known as 'Simmond's test' or 'Thompson's test'. (Interestingly, Simmond's described this test several years before but it is widely called the 'Thompson's test'.) This is a way of assessing the integrity of the tendon. The patient lies in the prone position on a bed, or kneels on a chair facing backwards, with their feet slightly hanging off the end. On squeezing the calf, a normal intact tendon will plantar-flex the foot. Absence of this movement suggests an Achilles tendon rupture. In any cases of uncertainty, an ultrasound scan or even MRI may aid the diagnosis.

ii. What drugs can weaken and therefore make an Achilles tendon rupture more likely?

There are several drugs implicated in an Achilles tendon rupture and it is a favourite question in examinations. Corticosteroids, especially-long term use, can potentiate a weakened tendon. Quinolones such as ciprofloxacin are a rarer cause, especially in the elderly. Rheumatoid arthritis and Cushing's are also associated with rupture.

iii. What treatment options are available?

The two main treatment approaches are conservative and surgical management, taking into consideration the patient's age, lifestyle and impact on quality of life. Conservative treatment involves a protocol of plaster cast and subsequent bracing with guided mobilization. Surgical treatment involves suture repair of the tendon. Outcomes of both have been shown to be comparable with effective rehabilitation and physiotherapy regimens.

OUTCOME

The patient opted for surgical management due to his high performance as a fighting athlete. Unfortunately, he suffered a re-rupture of the tendon after being hit in the wound by an arrow. This was complicated by a deep infection and he later died from wound sepsis. As his death came within 6 months of an operation, the coroner was informed. The inquest continues.

CASE 50

Casanova, a dashing Venetian, presents to your clinic complaining of a penile discharge. He reports that this has been going on now for several days. He is initially quite evasive but then explains that he has had multiple sexual partners in the past 4 weeks. On further questioning, he reports having intercourse with five ladies but is concerned as they are all married and he does not want their husbands to find out. On examination, he has a purulent discharge, is afebrile and otherwise has no significant past medical history. You swab the discharge and it comes back as a gram-negative diplococcus and you give him intramuscular ceftriaxone.

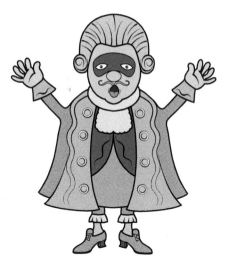

i. What is the likely diagnosis?

It is likely this patient has picked up a sexually transmitted infection, given his multiple partners and history of a discharge. It is likely he has gonorrhoea, given the gram-negative swab. There is increasing resistance of gonorrhoea to ciprofloxacin and cephalosporins are now more commonly used.

ii. To what other infection is this patient at risk?

A high proportion of patients with gonorrhoea will also have concurrent chlamydia infection and so this is often treated for at the same time. Chlamydia is the most common sexually transmitted infection in the UK and is often asymptomatic in both males and females, therefore a high index of suspicion is needed. It can cause issues later in life with infertility, epididymitis, pelvic inflammatory disease and a higher incidence of ectopic pregnancies being among the complications if left untreated.

iii. What is contact tracing?

It is often better for these patients to be seen in a Sexual Health clinic where they have access to counsellors and can contact trace. Contact tracing is the identification and follow up of a patient that has been infected. This helps reduce the spread of infection and also allows partners who may be asymptomatic to be treated, reducing disease burden and complications. The partners are informed that they should present for screening without naming the patient. It can be done anonymously and can raise some sensitive and ethical issues, and it is therefore helpful that the health advisors are trained and experienced in dealing with these difficult situations.

OUTCOME

Casanova was treated for gonorrhoea and also had a single dose of azithromycin to cover for the possible chlamydia infection. He was quite nervous about the contact tracing but, after discussion with the health advisors, provided the details of his partners. Despite this incident, he continued to liaise with married women, resulting in a few duels with some important people. He was denounced by the church as lacking in morals and later appeared on a Jerry Springer show entitled 'Who's your daddy?'

CASE 51

Cyclops presents to your clinic complaining of sudden painless visual
loss. He says this happened suddenly
and was like a curtain coming down
across the vision. He does not think
that there have been any foreign bodies entering his eye, although he had
been helping his friend Odysseus
move some sheep. He is normally fit
and well, although he does have a
diagnosis of hypertension. He does
not take any regular medications. On
examination, he reports being unable

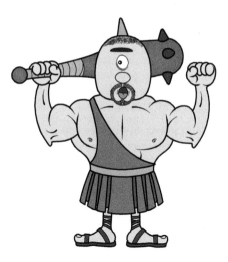

to see out of his eye and the visual acuity chart therefore cannot be completed. There are no obvious foreign bodies in the eye or under the eyelids.

i. How do you assess visual acuity?

Visual acuity is assessed using a standardized eye chart (Snellen chart; Fig. 51.1).
Patients stand 6 metres from the chart and read the letters. Normal vision is
reported as 6/6. If the reading is, for example, 6/60, this means a patient needs
to stand 6 metres away to see something the normal population could read from
60 metres.

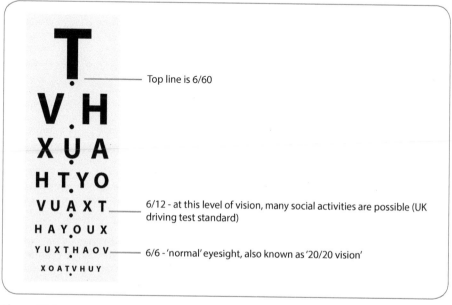

Figure 51.1.

ii. What is the differential of sudden visual loss?

Sudden visual loss is very distressing to a patient. A lot can be gained from the history to point you towards a diagnosis and patients will need to be seen urgently by an ophthalmologist. Listed below are some of the common causes of sudden PAINLESS loss of vision that you need to be aware of:

- **Ischaemic optic neuropathy** – (commonly results from temporal arteritis, also atherosclerosis). Clues in the history for temporal arteritis would be a headache, tenderness over the temporal artery, scalp tenderness or jaw claudication, and the condition is associated with polymyalgia rheumatica.
- **Vitreous haemorrhage.** Often in patients with diabetes or due to trauma. Mild haemorrhage may be characterized by floaters.
- **Occlusion of the central retinal vein.** In exams, the clue in the history is the presence of retinal haemorrhages.
- **Occlusion of the central retinal artery.** A 'cherry red' spot is classically seen on fundoscopy. There may be a pale retina around this due to the ischaemia, and it is often due to thromboembolism because of atherosclerosis.
- **Retinal detachment.** Often the history is one of a curtain or veil or dark shadow coming down over the eye. It can be seen on fundoscopy and may be preceded by floaters.

iii. What are the main serious causes of a red eye?

There are many causes of a red eye, with foreign body, dry eyes and conjunctivitis being the most common; a lot can be gleaned from the history. We have tried to describe below some of the distinguishing features that are often tested in exams:

- **Anterior uveitis.** This is often associated with ankylosing spondylitis. Patients will complain of acute onset of pain, blurred vision or photophobia, and on examination there may be a small and irregular fixed pupil.
- **Acute angle closure glaucoma.** Patients complain of severe pain (either eye pain or a headache), decreased visual acuity, a hazy cornea and semi-dilated pupils.
- **Scleritis.** This is associated with autoimmune diseases such as rheumatoid arthritis and is painful, often worse on movement. To differentiate between episcleritis and scleritis, the important difference is that episcleritis is not painful.
- **Episcleritis.** This is classically not painful and therefore distinguishes it from scleritis.

- **Foreign body**. This is often apparent in the history and it is important when assessing the eye to look under the upper eyelid. Fluorescein can also show corneal abrasions.
- **Conjunctivitis**. This can be viral or bacterial – often a clear discharge points towards a diagnosis of viral conjunctivitis.

OUTCOME

Cyclops was seen the same day by the ophthalmologist, who diagnosed retinal detachment. He underwent a vitrectomy, although his vision was slow to improve. He was unable to drive and this made him feel quite isolated from his friends and he fell out with Odysseus.

CASE 52

A gentleman with an eyepatch and a long black beard is brought into the department. His name is Blackbeard. He has been helicoptered in from a ship off shore when he started complaining of acutely painful left leg. His leg suddenly became cold and painful and feels numb to his touch. He has previously had a similar problem in his right leg and now wears a wooden prosthetic 'peg'. You examine the leg and find it to be pale and cold. You cannot feel any pulses in his foot; however, his radial pulse is fast and irregularly irregular. There is an ulcer present on the dorsum of the foot.

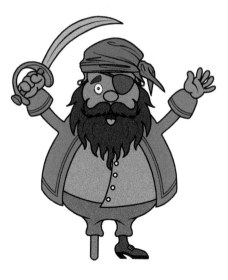

i. What are the causes of acute limb ischaemia?

There are three main causes: (1) thrombosis where an atheroma ruptures and thrombus forms on top of the plaque causing occlusion; (2) embolism where a thrombus travels from a proximal source such as heart mural thrombus in atrial fibrillation or post myocardial infarction, aortic aneurysm or prosthetic valve; and (3) trauma including compartment syndrome and dissection. The cardinal signs of acute limb ischaemia are best remembered as the 6 P's: pain, pallor, pulselessness, paraesthesia, perishingly cold, paralysis.

ii. What is Virchow's triad?

This states that any of the three components can lead to thrombosis within a vessel (Fig. 52.1). Stasis can be caused by immobility, atrial fibrillation or

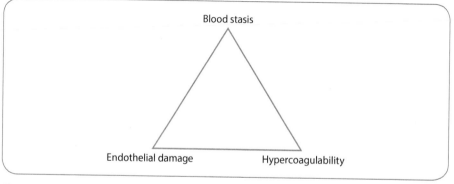

Figure 52.1.

extrinsic vessel compression; endothelial damage can be caused by trauma, prosthetic material, hypertension or atherosclerosis; hypercoagulability can be caused by dehydration, active cancer, obesity or clotting disorders.

iii. How do you differentiate between the types of ulcers?

The three main types of ulcers are arterial, venous and neuropathic. More rarely they can be caused by trauma, infection or malignancy. Distinguishing features are shown in the table below (Fig. 52.2).

	Venous	Arterial	Neuropathic
History	Aching and swelling worse at the end of the day, relieved by elevation, Previous varicose veins or DVT	Pain after exertion or leg elevation. History of smoking or peripheral vascular disease	Numbness, burning or paraesthesia in the foot. History of diabetes or peripheral neuropathy
Location	Gaiter area between medial malleolus and calf	Distally (e.g. toes)	Pressure areas (e.g. heel, metatarsal heads)
Ulcer bed	Granulating base with exudate	Dry necrotic base	Variable depth with possible exposure of underlying tendon or bone
Appearance	Shallow irregular margins with sloping edges.	Deep and punched out with well-defined border	Surrounding callus, may be sinus tract indicating osteomyelitis
Surrounding skin	Haemosiderin deposits and Epodermatosclerosis	Cool, pale, hair loss with weak pulses (ABPI <0.9)	Insensate and often calloused
Management	Leg elevation and compression bandaging	Smoking cessation, antiplatelets and revascularization	Diabetic control, chiropody and debridement of necrotic tissue

Figure 52.2.

OUTCOME

Blackbeard was found to be in atrial fibrillation and to have an embolus in the superficial femoral artery. After urgent femoral embolectomy his foot perfusion improved and his ulcers healed. He required a lengthy review of his social situation, but after fitting of hand-rails on the top deck, a toilet seat rise in the heads and stocking the galley full of ready meals he was able to return to swashbuckling on the high seas.

Index